GIRLISH

THE ULTIMATE HANDBOOK ON PUBERTY FOR GIRLS
AGED 9 TO 12

LONDON FORD

CONTENTS

JUST FOR YOU

A FREE GIFT TO OUR READERS
A Period-Penning Journal book to remember all your
thoughts and actions with fun pictures that will help
you through your growth journey.

Send an email to:
londonfordbooks@yahoo.com

INTRODUCTION

Being a girl is fun and all until we face the little changes and annoyances that make us feel all alone and *different.* But the truth is, although no two girls will face the exact same cycles, symptoms, and timeframe of maturity, we all have one thing in common: Our bodies will change and grow. Moreover, we all will have our periods one day, if we haven't already. The key is to know and understand that this is natural, manageable, and—despite what we might think—something we can live with for decades without dying of embarrassment, cramps, or any of the other irritants that come with our period.

Menstruation is frequently still a touchy issue and, in some cases, considered taboo. But this should not be so. Even in school health classes that cover the topic, the emphasis is sometimes placed on the fundamentals without ever mentioning the actual real experience of a monthly cycle, so whatever advice girls do hear around them can be unfavorable or misleading. Your first menstruation may, therefore, be unsettling.

However, you can learn to face your menstrual cycle in a completely different way by learning lots of factual knowledge, hearing about real-life experiences, and getting useful advice as a key indicator of approaching adulthood.

Speaking of female nature, it turns out that only a small number of animals on Earth, including humans, have females that experience menstruation. Only five other animals in the animal kingdom have a menstrual cycle, making it an unusual occurrence (EUSci, 2020). Some might even say it's a special occurrence. Though the animal cycle might be different, this indicates that the uniqueness of this naturally occurring cycle is a scientifically amazing phenomenon that should be free of any social stigma.

I carefully considered every aspect of this book before putting it together to create the best handbook for girls going through puberty. We must normalize the conversation surrounding periods, and the first step in doing so is learning more about our bodies and how they function throughout this time. Girls today are maturing at a young age, thus you should be better prepared to manage these situations. So, it makes sense that I would want to write a book to share everything I've learned with my readers.

Expect interesting, useful, and original advice and information from these seven chapters that will certainly make you smile. Remember to relax because this book is just meant to be helpful; as a result, each lesson is delivered in an approachable and pleasurable way so that you can enjoy reading it.

1

EMOTIONS IN YOUR BRAIN

Girls aren't new to emotions. Many times we've felt sad if our pet died or happy when the teacher suggests a new game in class. But rarely have we ever had to *understand* our emotions, right? The more we grow, the more we realize that we simply... can't. We might think we understand, but it still can be pretty hard to interpret the emotions swirling around in our brains and hearts.

The truth is, as we grow and the big Momma P (puberty) invades our lives, we will start to see changes in our emotions, often unwanted and confusing, and most of the time they are linked with our periods. The bottom line is that we understand that it does happen, and it is one hundred percent normal.

Tweens—young people from the ages of 9 to 12—frequently experience mixed emotions that range from upbeat and joyful to weary, flat, or melancholy. Tweens frequently need more privacy or alone time, which is completely acceptable and normal. These emotional ups and downs can occur more frequently and to a greater degree during this period of your life.

Physical, social, and emotional factors can all play a role in your fluctuating feelings; no single factor alone is to blame. You might frequently notice that you aren't able to pinpoint the exact cause of how you are feeling. And again, that is completely fine. Here, I'll tell you how to control, understand, and deal with these emotional ups, downs, crisses, and crosses.

GROWING UP: EMOTIONS AND ADOLESCENCE

Moods are a sign that you are dealing with more sophisticated, mature emotions and are making an effort to comprehend and control them. This is a critical stage in adolescent development.

It sounds funny to say, but feelings are too significant to get upset over. They are a great source of information about ourselves. Our ability to feel is a crucial tool for self-awareness just like our abilities to see, hear, smell, touch, discern, and think. Similar to how being blind or deaf is partially disabling, being disconnected from or out of touch with our emotions can also be partially disabling because essential communication with ourselves is lacking. And trust me, the last thing you want is to be lacking in communication with yourself. Why?

Because young teens have the potential for advanced thinking that might cause worry about the future. Preteens and teens may be overly concerned with

- academic progress
- physical development, popularity, and appearance
- the potential passing of a parent
- getting harassed in school
- school aggression
- lacking friends
- alcohol and drug use
- their parents' divorce
- their own mortality

That's a lot, isn't it? Perhaps you've thought about one or two of these things, or maybe even all of them. But the truth is, we all have different thoughts and we deal with them differently based on our emotions. This is why emotions need to be embraced, not shunned.

Though it might seem frustrating at times because we might not always understand them, it's okay to take these feelings by the horns and rein them in or, if needed, let them rage crazily. Anything you need.

Remember, it's easy to generalize emotions, especially by age, sex, family situation, or life in general. But in the end, they are *your* emotions, after all, so do what's best for you. Don't know how?

Let me show you.

Getting Through the Ups and Down

As a young teen, you might tend to be extremely self-conscious. And hey, it's okay. Most young adolescents experiment with various means of expressing their emotions in addition to the regular changes in the feelings they experience. For instance, a young child who enthusiastically greeted friends and family with a hug and a kiss may develop into a teenager who just waves or nods at them. The changes will soon become evident and maybe even hard to deal with, and here is born the era of emotional ups and downs. They may happen due to physical, social, and mental factors, but the fact still remains that they will happen. You just have to know how to manage and embrace them.

How to Manage Them

You will inevitably experience low or melancholy moods. First, you must understand that emotional ups and downs are normal and that you are not alone in experiencing them. I know it can be a scary and lonely time, especially if you don't have siblings around your age or have parents who "don't understand." But knowing that we all experience hard spots from time to time is one of the finest and first methods to manage your emotions.

Additionally, I know a lot of girls don't want to hear this, but wouldn't it be comforting to know that your parents and family around you have been through the same thing? Seems impossible, right? But they have. And another big secret that they probably won't tell you is that it might've been even harder for them! With technological advancement and easier access to (literally) everything, it's easier for girls today to keep parents, teachers, family, and friends at arm's length.

If you think they won't understand, just give it a try. When they come to you, don't shut them out. In contrast, you can go to them as well. Whether it's your mom, sister, aunt, guardian, school teacher, guidance counselor, or the sweet waiter at your family's favorite restaurant (as long as it is not a stranger!), there's someone who understands and someone who will help.

It might seem like a lot, but just take a shot and see where it goes. I'm your personal cheerleader!

Of course, it's okay if you need space. At this stage of becoming a woman, you are learning independence and solving problems on your own. It's a life skill that you will need to develop sooner or later. Problem-solving is an essential life skill and you will only get better at it by practicing!

You can also find coping strategies. One of the major tasks of adolescence is learning to deal with and regulate emotional ups and downs on your own. Of course, parents, loved ones, teachers, and even this book can help, but you will only benefit if you learn your own coping strategies because what works for me might not be what works for you.

Making a list of "mood busters" is one method to do this. You can do these tasks to feel better and manage your emotions and mood swings. Some examples of mood busters are

- listening to a happy song or your favorite music
- taking a little walk
- playing with or cuddling with pets
- receiving a hug
- playing games
- watching soothing videos

- reading
- talking
- dancing to favorite or upbeat music

Go ahead! Try a few options from the list to experiment with. Try out several ideas to discover what works best.

So, let's review. The first step in managing your emotions is accepting that they are normal and that you are not alone. We should also always have someone to lean on for grown-up advice and guidance. We might be growing up, but we still need others, especially those who have been through it all before and know how to help. Finally, you can find coping strategies to help keep your emotions balanced. You may need to experiment to find what works for you. Try to keep up with your activities. It'll help you feel secure and grounded and pave the way for new interests. Trust me, adolescence will bring a lot of new interests.

So be excited! This is a beautiful journey you are embarking on as a young woman. You'll have mood swings and pain sometimes, of course, but that shouldn't and won't take away from the beautiful moments of growing up!

Emotional changes can be annoying (like no-WiFi-level annoying), but that's okay! You know why? Because if you feel strange about your bodily and emotional changes, that means you're doing it right.

WHY IT'S DIFFERENT FOR BOYS

Do you know a boy your age? Is he going through the same things you are? Maybe your answer is no simply because we really don't take notice of emotional changes when it comes to our guy friends, right? Or maybe, at this stage of your life, boys are annoying and they don't seem to understand. Or perhaps you're having a strange feeling towards a certain someone that you don't understand, so he just seems rather annoying. Am I getting this right?

The truth is, they are going through it, too, whether we see it or not. It just might seem a little different. And here's why.

Male and female tweens often manage emotions quite differently, which is likely due to the same-sex socialization with peers that we experienced as children (girls are frequently encouraged to be sensitive and open about their feelings while boys are frequently encouraged to be strong and silent about their feelings).

Compared to boys, who can be more accustomed to repressing their feelings, girls seem more practiced at and used to expressing their emotions openly. This distinction need not exist if all adolescents, whether male or female, are educated at home that expressing one's emotions is acceptable and beneficial.

WHAT'S GOING ON IN MY BRAIN?

By now, we've established that a lot is happening in our minds at this age as girls. We hear that it's because we are growing up and changes are happening, but why exactly are these changes taking place? What is going on in our minds and bodies that is causing these changes?

Well, it happens because of puberty, and puberty happens because of hormones. And before you get all grossed out, there are many types of hormones all with different jobs. Let's take a moment to look at the science behind it.

Your brain cells become attached to hormones. A brain cell is differentiated from cells in other parts of the body because they have protruding portions that resemble wires. A brain cell normally has a lot of dendrites, which are smaller "wires," for receiving signals from neighboring cells. Additionally, some cells have a longer "wire" called an axon that communicates with other cells. Your brain cells can be affected by hormones in two different ways.

First, hormones can modify how the brain is structured, although these changes take time to happen. Second, a hormone may affect how brain cells respond to an event or environment by being activated. The ability of a cell to exchange messages with neighboring cells may be aided or hindered by hormones. Brain cells may also experience long-term changes as a result of this. Since the brain is still developing and hormone levels throughout puberty are higher than during childhood, this process is particularly crucial.

To summarize in simpler words, hormones work together with brain cells in puberty to develop teenage emotions and boost emotional maturity. As harsh as it might sound, it's their job, and without them, we wouldn't have the capacity to grow up and become emotionally mature.

What Growing Up Means to Your Brain

Some things can be learned more effectively by children than by teenagers or adults. But the fun part is that puberty might create an opportunity for different kinds of learning. It can present chances for self-discovery and the development of social and emotional competencies that help teenagers prepare for adulthood. Teenage years may bring about changes in the brain that enable such learning. For instance, responding to feedback—or how your brain processes information notifying you whether or not you have provided the correct answer—is a crucial component of learning new abilities.

Another crucial aspect of learning new skills is needing to experiment and take chances, such as talking to someone you like or trying out a new interest that you might not be very good at. When you believe there's something to gain, you might be more inclined to decide to take a risk.

You may be inspired to learn more about yourself and others as a result, promoting self-discovery and personal development. Because of where your brain is in the development process, you are more prone to

- act impulsively
- mistakenly perceive or misjudge social cues and emotions
- get into accidents of various types
- engage in conflict
- engage in unsafe or harmful actions

Teenagers are less inclined to

- think before acting
- pause to reflect on the effects of their actions
- alter their risky or harmful behaviors

Of course, this doesn't mean you can't still make wise decisions and discern right from wrong despite these brain changes due to hormones and puberty. Additionally, it does not free you of responsibility for your deeds. So, what was the point of this entire section?

It was to show you that not only will your emotions change, but your entire thought process will, too. It's good to be informed because when it happens, or if you're currently living through this, you will know how to tackle everything.

Always remember knowledge is power, and we are powerful ladies!

Other Changes in Your Brain

It is finally safe to say we can blame everything on our brains. Though it is one of the most important parts of our human body system, it can also be the most confusing part in terms of what messages it is sending our bodies.

The thing about growing up is that your mind is in a constant battle with pushing past childhood and moving into adolescence, so it is experimenting with a variety of things to determine what kind of teenager, and eventually adult, you will become. When these things start to happen, there's no need to worry. As crazy and confusing as it is, it's normal, and it's all our brain's fault. So, here are just a few things that happen in your brain that cause changes in your body, moods, attitudes, and interactions. I'll just leave a few so when they actually start to happen (or perhaps they already have), you won't be too alarmed and you'll know that these things are just as natural as breathing.

Heightened Sensitivity

Since your body changes so much during puberty, it's normal to feel uncomfortable about them and become overly self-conscious about how you look. As a result, you can become easily annoyed, snap at people, or experience depression. It will be beneficial to be conscious of the behavioral changes you have under-gone and to discuss them with someone you trust.

Seeking Identity

Since you're in the process of maturing into an adult, you might feel compelled to discover what makes you special. Additionally, there is a typical inclination for you to associate with your friends more than your family. It can be psychologically related to the fact that you and your friends are experiencing the same stage of life. You might try to determine how you are unique from other people and where you belong in the world. This can eventually result in a struggle to distance yourself from your parents and other family members.

Contrasting Ideas

You could feel trapped between who you were as a child and who you want to be as an adult because, as a tween or teenager going through puberty, you are in a transitional stage. For instance, you might wish to be more independent while simultaneously needing to look to your parents for assistance. A different example is whether you want to give up your childhood interests in order to fit in with your peers. You can feel conflicted as a result and seek clarification.

Feeling Unsure

Puberty can potentially result in uncertain times because you're neither fully an adult nor a child anymore. You might start to ponder and consider new and unknown parts of life, such as a career, a means of livelihood, and relationships, during this transitional period. When you start thinking in these terms, everything is fresh and strange, therefore you might feel unsure about the future.

When the expectations that those close to you have of you also change, this uncertainty is more obvious. Greater obligations than those placed on you as a child might now be demanded of you. You will eventually settle into your new position and gain more self-assurance, but this process could take time.

Mood Swings

You might also suffer frequent and even significant fluctuations in mood in addition to confused and conflicting emotions. For instance, sometimes in a short period of time, your mood will change from feeling satisfied and pleased to feeling irritated and dejected. Mood swings are abrupt changes in your emotional state. They could be brought on by your body's fluctuating hormone levels or other puberty-related changes.

Peer Pressure

Your interactions with your peers will become more frequent as puberty approaches. What you observe around you in popular media and the culture that is reflected there is likely to have an impact on you and your social circle. Depending on what you see, you might frequently grab on to what's trendy in terms of how you speak, dress, and even act.

This could be awkward and uncomfortable and might even alter your preferences. Additionally, it's one of the reasons you might encounter difficulty fitting in with your peers. These incidents may cause a difference between what your friends and parents deem suitable.

Sensing Self-Consciousness

Every person experiences puberty at a different time. As a result, your growth may differ from that of your peers. You may become more aware of your body and the way you're developing as a result.

Because girls mature earlier and more quickly than boys, these experiences are more evident in girls. Additionally, their physical changes—like the enlargement of their hips and the development of their breasts—are more obvious. The presence of their classmates who are in the same age bracket could make them feel self-conscious about their bodies.

Cognitive Changes

Although they may be harder to notice, early adolescent cognitive (your ability to process and access knowledge and understanding) and mental changes can be equally as important as those that occur physically and emotionally. Most adolescents undergo major mental, logical, and academic growth during adolescence.

In order to be convinced that something is genuine, younger children need to see and touch it. However, as tweens and teenagers, we start to develop the ability to think independently and about more abstract things that we can't see or feel. You improve your ability to analyze issues and consider the effects of various view-points or actions.

It's also a fun fact that young teens are able to acquire more difficult and complex information in school thanks to these cognitive changes. So, that means you will develop an eagerness to learn, apply what you learn, and think through various choices. Your emotional life is also affected by these mental changes. For instance, your ability to reason may affect how you interact with and behave around your parents. You might start to prepare an explanation or an answer in anticipation of your parents' reactions to something you have said or done. Admit it, hasn't there been a time—at least one—where you made a decision based on what you believe your parents might say or do? It's pretty much due to these mental changes.

You will also be prompted by these mental changes to reflect on who you are and who you might become. This is what we call identity formation. It's a process that occurs during adolescence and is important for your growth.

The majority of your peers will experiment with many identities. You will all go through "phases," which can seem to parents and grown-ups to be constantly chang-ing. In fact, teenagers who skip this phase of exploring are more likely to experience mental issues as adults, especially despair. So, if you are going through a phase, even though you might not see it as such, don't be afraid to explore it, no matter how odd or hard it is.

Similar to how adults with more life experience and brain development can struggle with their various roles, teenagers also have trouble coming to terms with who they are. Sometimes you might feel like a different person based on who you are interacting with. It's your mind's way of adapting to your environment and situation so it can pick and choose what it likes or doesn't, and in turn, forms your true identity.

But don't rush or force it. It will take years before you're at the level of full maturity. Your only job is to keep on the right track and ensure your friends and role models are leading you down the right path. The trick to knowing if you're on the right path is asking yourself this: Would you show this to or talk about it with your parents?

If the answer is a big fat NO, then you might want to reconsider your decisions.

Although young teens might well be capable of thinking more maturely, you still lack the life experience necessary to act as such in every instance. As a result, sometimes actions might not match your beliefs.

In the end, young teens and their parents need some time to get used to all these changes. But there is also excitement in the changes. They enable you to envision your potential and make preparations to become that person.

And I know that whoever you become will be extraordinary.

THERE ARE NO BAD EMOTIONS

Despite the fact that emotions are neither good nor bad, individuals frequently categorize them according to how they are felt.

Therefore, "good" emotions could include

- pleasure
- love
- joy
- excitement
- appreciation

People enjoy feeling these and other good emotions in general.

On the other hand, "bad" emotions could include

- fear
- sadness
- anger
- irritation
- jealousy

These and other unfavorable emotions are generally unpleasant for people to feel.

But is this really so? Or is it simply the way we perceive it?

Now comes the challenging part for teenagers. Teenagers are particularly vulnerable to the effects of emotions. The entire stigma of good or bad emotions is how they are interpreted and the messages they send and, in turn, the resulting actions. This means that the mental choice is left up to the emotional state. Take a look at a few typical examples:

- In order to improve situations, **discouragement** may advise you to look at the negative rather than the positive.
- **Anger** can encourage backlash rather than addressing the issue in a way that will improve the situation.

- Instead of facing the issue head-on and taking action to improve the situation, **fear** may advise running away.
- **Helplessness** may encourage giving up rather than continuing to work toward improvement.
- Being **lonely** can encourage further isolation as opposed to reaching out to improve circumstances.
- **Insecurity** may advise you to remain silent rather than speak up to improve the situation.
- **Shame** might advise you to stay hidden rather than openly talk to improve the situation.
- Instead of taking action to improve the situation on your own behalf, **depression** may force you to remain inactive.

But here's the advice you ought to listen to in order to bust the myth of "bad" emotions: When it comes to managing emotions, use them to get informed and become emotionally stronger and more intelligent, but also use your reasoning to figure out what's best to do. Of course, emotions can be negative, but the reactions and results do not have to be, and that, really, is the line between what makes it good and bad. What you do with your emotions matters.

Girls, Here's the Truth

Our world is not known for being emotionally accepting. Emotions can be quite loud, after all, so it can be difficult and messy to deal with them.

The likelihood is that, as a young and growing woman, you are affected by these mixed signals of emotions in a variety of ways.

But if we look around us, this constant pressure of emotions doesn't seem to be thrown on boys as much, does it? And girls are always being told how to deal with emotions and what to do if we feel a certain way. Because of the general stereotype smacked on us from the beginning of time, we have been shaped in such a way as to portray the more emotional beings of our species.

Yep. That's deep.

This is not to say that we can't feel emotions, or if we do, that we should act all tough and closed-off as most boys your age might. No. We are to embrace and be comfortable with our emotions and never be afraid to talk about them. Shout it from the mountain tops, if you please.

The focus is to know that there is *nothing* wrong with being emotional and that it doesn't make you "girly," "a cry baby," "whiny," or "annoying." It just makes you human.

However, females learn early that complex emotions like anger and jealousy seem to be taboo and are seen negatively by adults. As a result, we develop habits of denying and ignoring our feelings which can put girls at risk for anxiety and depression.

Girls are much more prone than boys to experience anxiety disorders, and they experience depression at rates that are twice as high in adolescence (Pruess, 2018). Still, this has nothing whatsoever to do with being "too" emotional.

So what is the secret to keeping ourselves from going down the rabbit hole of anxiety and depression?

Emotional intelligence.

Though we will talk more about emotional intelligence later, here's what we're focusing on now: Once we are able to comprehend and control our emotions, we can begin to establish the foundation for emotional maturity and effective coping skills.

You might've learned to handle certain emotions from a young age by being exposed to coping techniques that help you to endure waves of intense emotions. We are less likely to use unhealthy coping mechanisms, such as overeating, self-harming, or abusing drugs, when we have the skills to handle problems and access a variety of good coping strategies. This is the beginning of controlling your emotions and developing emotional intelligence.

Whatever calms and soothes your body, mind, and emotions can be added to this inexhaustive list of coping and relaxing techniques:

- using headphones to listen to music (not too loud!)
- journaling
- creating art in your own way
- reading something you love
- keeping stuffed animals or soft blankets
- using fidgets or stress balls
- drinking warm liquids, having a warm bath, or using a heating pad
- taking a moment of silence alone
- talking with friends and loved ones
- exercising
- joining an extracurricular activity that you love

Have you ever watched a teen movie where the female lead has a journal or diary or is always reading, has a best friend who she can talk to about anything, and enjoys a certain hobby to calm herself down? Well, there you have it. It can be just the same in your life. You just have to find what works best for you.

Building Your Emotional Intelligence

Wait! Before you groan and say this sounds boring, just hear me out. Wouldn't it be awesome to have a superpower? And perhaps we won't be flying or shooting lasers from our eyes anytime soon, but what if we could control the biggest superpower of them all? The female mind.

Sounds cool, right?

What if it was a power that would improve decision-making with intelligence and kindness, decrease or eliminate violence, instill in people a desire for kindness and compassion, and build connections that unite, heal, nourish, and allow people to flourish? Well, if every adolescent on the earth learned emotional intelligence, we could accomplish this, and it could change our way of life in so many ways. I don't know about you, but I think that's a pretty awesome superpower.

The fact is, not every teenager needs to know this. Only you.

Knowing what other people actually feel and being able to recognize and correctly manage our own emotions and relationships are both elements of emotional intelligence. Your chances of succeeding in school and in life will increase if you develop social and emotional intelligence. Below are a few ways you can achieve this.

Be Real and Human

Own your humanity—it is lovely, and no one else on Earth does humanity quite like you do. It's fine to make mistakes and fail, so be kind to yourself when it happens. You'll experience bad days and bad moments, and occasionally, you'll make errors. It is a core part of interacting, growing, and existing as an adolescent.

Be Kind

The foundation of human relationships, social skills, and connection is kindness. Being told to be kind is one thing, but practicing kindness toward yourself, your friends, your siblings and parents, and even strangers is where the magic lies.

Learn How to Listen

To be lovable, you must learn to listen. Hearing is not the same as listening. Take time to listen to others and try to give constructive advice as best as you can. This will help you to mature because you learn from others by listening, too, whether it's someone older than you, a television program, or your peers.

Empathy

Empathy—or being able to understand what someone's going through and be supportive and kind—is an essential life skill and is necessary for healthy relationships and emotional growth. Talk to your parents or a friend about a problem that they are having and practice being understanding and supportive by putting yourself in their shoes. You will have firsthand knowledge of the impact empathy has.

Healthy Disagreements

Maintaining relationships and developing a sense of identity in those relationships requires being able to successfully negotiate different viewpoints. It's fine to occasionally disagree with your parents or peers, but keep an open mind regarding their perspectives. You don't have to agree with someone to understand them. It shows your respect for their right to an opinion as well as your desire to maintain the relationship and the conversation. Even if you disagree, people will always respect others who respect their opinions.

Share Your Emotions

It's important to keep in mind that everyone experiences sadness, anger, fear, jealousy, and insecurity. When appropriate, express your feelings to others. Keeping your emotions to yourself won't make them go away. Picture it like this: It's like piling rocks on a piece of glass until the glass finally cracks. It's always good to talk and express your feelings with someone you can trust.

Relationships Are Essential

Whether it's with your cat, a friend, or a family member, maintaining relationships is important for emotional growth and intelligence. Even if you are the most introverted person, you are not an island, and you can't face everything alone. So, even if you feel a pull away from your family as you grow up, continue to work to maintain or build a relationship with them. At some point in your rapid ascent to adulthood, you're going to need someone, and the best people are those who love you the most, so hold onto those people. You're going to need them, and when they need you, ensure you are always there.

What Emotions Do

Every emotion has a significant reason for existing:

- Anger gives us the drive to make things right and is a sign that something is wrong.
- Sadness causes us to temporarily withdraw from the outside world in order to reset,

recharge, and recover. It also signals to others that we might need some caring.

- When we are afraid, we have the strength and stamina to either fight or run away from a harmful situation.
- Anxiety motivates us to respond to a possible threat. (If it can be reframed as "excitement" when it pertains to a performance, it can work for, rather than against, the performance).
- Jealousy alerts us to vital matters and directs our attention to potential areas for development.
- When we have negative feelings about a friendship, it may be a sign that the friendship isn't a good one for us to be in, that we deserve more, or that it's time to let go.

Paying attention to the feeling will provide hints as to what is required to find balance. Identify the words or signals that are associated with the emotion. It doesn't matter if there aren't any; what matters is that you are developing your ability for self-awareness, emotional awareness, and awareness of your needs.

Remember, you don't have to do this alone. Reach out to a role model or your parents while developing your emotional intelligence as it is a vital part of your development as a tween and teen.

PERIOD PENNINGS

Let's reflect!

Take this section to write about how you feel about your emotions, what has changed, and what you will do from now on to try and control and embrace your emotions.

Ponder these questions:

1. Do you think your hormones have changed your body, mind, and emotions in any way? If so, how?
2. Will you be able to embrace the changes in your emotions, mood swings, and the overall effect of puberty?
3. What else do you anticipate to change soon?

_____
_____
_____
_____
_____
_____
_____
_____
_____
_____
_____

Segue: The next chapter explains puberty.

WHAT IS PUBERTY?

Remember when you couldn't wait to grow up? Now you are growing up, and before you reach the destination, you will have to go through your adolescence. Adolescence is right around the corner for you, but there's a small station that you need to stop at first—the station of puberty.

WHAT IS PUBERTY?

In theory, the period of time when your body starts to alter and develop as you transition from a child to an adult is known as puberty. We're talking about things like boys growing facial hair and girls getting breasts. With the exception of when you were a baby, your body will grow more quickly during adolescence than any other time in your life.

When a person reaches puberty, they begin to sexually mature. It's a phase that typically takes place between the ages of 12 and 16 for boys and 10 and 14 for girls. It results in bodily changes and has varied effects on boys and girls.

Puberty, which occurs in the first few years of adolescence, is a normal stage of development. Though there are many additional—and sometimes embarrassing—physical changes associated with puberty, such as hair growth, body odor, and pimples, do you know what exactly occurs in your body during this time? As we discussed earlier, the brain sends instructions in the form of hormones to the body to mark the beginning of puberty.

All of your body's primary organs and systems mature during puberty. At the end of puberty, you will be reproductively mature. This is why girls get their periods during puberty. If you haven't gotten your period yet, there's a high chance that it's on its way and will find you in the next few years. This is not something to worry about or be scared of. We will talk about everything (and I mean everything) about periods later. But, in general, changes in your body's hormone levels during puberty are what cause the growth and development that takes place.

The emotional changes discussed earlier are all due to puberty, too.

This is to say that so much happens in this relatively brief stage of your life.

It is important to be aware of the changes that puberty brings about so you can be prepared. Additionally, it's critical to keep in mind that everyone experiences these changes. You will encounter them regardless of your location, gender, or if you're a cereal-then-milk or milk-then-cereal person.

Although no two individuals are alike in every way, puberty is a shared experience for all of us.

Your pituitary gland, a pea-shaped gland found at the base of your brain, releases specific hormones when your body is prepared to start the puberty process. These hormones affect various areas of the body depending on if you're a boy or a girl.

In girls, puberty is usually accompanied by the following experiences:

- Typically, the growth of breasts is the first sign of puberty. The beginning of breast development is referred to as "budding." The breasts can occasionally vary in size. During this time, the breasts may feel sensitive.
- Your pubic region and armpits will then experience hair growth, and the hair on your arms and legs will begin to darken.
- Periods, or menstruation, typically join the party soon after. Periods are a natural aspect of the monthly cycle in which the lining of the uterus (womb) thickens to prepare the body for reproduction. If pregnancy has not occurred, the lining is lost over a few days once a month. Even though periods follow a cycle, in the first stages of puberty, the length of the cycle varies from month to month.
- Your body will become curvier and your hips will broaden.
- You'll grow taller. Height will vary for girls based on genes, age, and other factors. With all of this rapid growth, it could appear that one area of your body, like your feet, is developing more rapidly than the rest. You might feel awkward or clumsy as a result. This is also normal. Eventually, the rest of your body will catch up and fill out, and you'll feel less clumsy.

- You might experience acne. This is a skin condition that appears as bumps usually found on the chest, upper back, shoulders, and face. These bumps could be cysts, pimples, blackheads, or whiteheads. Teenagers with acne experience hormonal changes during puberty.
- Just prior to or at the beginning of your period, you may begin to experience pain or cramps.

Physical changes aren't the only things that puberty brings into your once-simple life. It also brings social, cognitive, and emotional changes. Your mood and feelings may be affected by things like

- hormones
- sleep deprivation
- peer pressure
- demands of school
- trouble with family
- feelings of fear or isolation
- stress
- anxiety
- a packed schedule
- feeling embarrassed or self-conscious
- higher decision-making abilities

This might be a lot to process since puberty isn't courteous enough to ask if we are ready. But it will be easier once you are informed, so don't ever be afraid to research, read more, and ask questions! It will make the process much easier.

WHAT TRIGGERS PUBERTY?

Let's talk about science for a moment. It'll be fun!

Our genes work in the body like different musical melodies that are combined to create your body's unique song. As we learned earlier, special compounds called hormones act as conductors that are produced in specific body regions and travel through the blood to instruct other parts of the body on what to do when the time is right. The various organ systems that make up the human body are like the tools that follow the conductor's instructions and bring the whole thing to life. Hormones act as messengers that move throughout the body during these complex times of transition, giving instructions to grow (or stop growing), change size and shape, or produce more (or less) of something that your body requires. Hormones control the whole reproductive system, including puberty.

For females, the following factors determine when puberty begins:

- **Weight**: Sometimes a girl with a higher body weight might enter puberty earlier.
- **Nutrition**: Puberty can be delayed if a girl isn't getting the nutrition her body needs.
- **Genetics**: Daughters of moms who experienced early puberty are more likely to experience it as well.
- **Ethnicity**: Puberty typically begins earlier in Black and Hispanic girls than in Asian and White girls who are not also Hispanic.

When your brain releases the hormones responsible for puberty, a special hormone called estrogen is then released by the ovaries which helps the development of the reproductive system and your changing characteristics. Now here's the tricky part: The release of gonadotropin-releasing hormone (GnRH) from the hypothalamus (a region of the brain that controls hormones) is what causes puberty in both males and females.

Two hormones—luteinizing hormone (LH) and follicle-stimulating hormone (FSH)—are released by the pituitary gland in response to this hormone (GnRH). These hormones activate the process leading to sexual maturity by traveling through the blood to your ovaries (BBC, 2014).

I don't intend for you to grasp everything in just one reading, but in essence, the numerous changes that take place during puberty are due to shifting hormone levels.

There are two key hormones involved in puberty that don't necessarily deal with your reproductive system:

- **Growth hormone**: The levels of this rise throughout puberty, resulting in a rapid increase in height accompanied by growth spurts in your bones and muscles.
- **Estradiol**: Both males and females have this. Estradiol levels in females increase earlier and stay higher after puberty.

Thus, all these new chemicals are flowing around inside your body during puberty, transforming you from a tween to an adolescent with higher levels of hormones.

Progesterone and Estrogen

Essential hormones in the formation of adolescent reproductive function include progesterone and estrogen. During puberty, both hormone levels rise dramatically, which causes the body to go through a lot of changes.

During the second half of the menstrual cycle, progesterone primarily affects the uterus to prepare it for
pregnancy (though we are far away from that stage).
Still, in order to enable the implantation of a fertilized
egg, it thickens the uterus's lining. This lining falls away
if pregnancy does not take place and is released as a
menstrual flow. We'll touch more on periods in later
chapters, but this is the role of the progesterone
hormone.

The majority of the other puberty-related alterations
are induced by estrogens.

Estrogen has the ability to transform female sexual
organs from those of a kid into those of an adult,
among other effects. It promotes the development of
the uterus, fallopian tubes, vagina, and ovaries. The
labia majora and minora, which are part of the external
genitalia, also enlarge.

The growth of the breasts is also a result of estrogen.
More fat is accumulated there as well as the formation
of a vast stretchy system. Estrogen's influence also
contributes to the capacity for milk production.

Estrogens prevent bone from being reabsorbed. Due to
bone expansion, female puberty height growth is rapid
for many years. However, estrogens also force the
bones to stop developing sooner in females than in

males, so most of the time, females stop growing sooner than males. Cool, isn't it?

As a result, women are typically shorter than men.

Still, women have a larger amount of body fat than men because estrogens promote the development of fatty tissue. Particularly, fat accumulates in the breasts, thighs, hips, and buttocks. The result is the recognizable feminine "hourglass" form. Female skin thickens as well, although it is still thinner, softer, and warmer than male skin of the same age.

The reality is that every girl won't have the same body shape, height, and composition. This doesn't mean your estrogen is faulty or "not working." It just means we are all special, unique, and beautiful in our own ways, and when we finally get our adult bodies at twenty-something years old, we should love and cherish everything about it.

Because we are all awesome.

How Can You Hit Puberty? And Does It Hit Back?

Puberty definitely hits like a smack to the face. Without much of a warning and in the most confusing ways, puberty can and will hit you and change almost everything about your childhood. So, how do you hit it back?

The key to hitting back is first embracing and accepting that puberty needs to happen and we just have to go through it. Rejecting, resisting, and fighting it will only result in stress, frustration, emotions all over the place, and unwanted struggles. So, hold it by the reins and drive your own way into adulthood instead of being plunged into it. This section talks about how to do just that.

Welcome Your Body's Changes

Don't fight the changes taking place in your body; they are beneficial. The normal transition to adulthood is often overlooked in Western societies which have a tendency to shame any sort of weight increase. Instead of feeling the desperate need to control them, try to observe these changes with a grateful awareness. Your mental strain will be greatly reduced when you feel connected to your body, which will free you up to concentrate on other crucial matters.

Know That Everything Changes

Your brain is significantly affected by rising hormones, which makes it much simpler to focus on small details. Remember that everything passes. If you ever feel over-burdened at school, home, or with friends, go for a walk outside and take some deep breaths.

Keep a Journal

Write down your ideas, emotions, and even little details about your day. Avoid tearing out and tearing up the pages. Save them; someday you'll be so glad you did. Reading about your own development in the pages of your journals will bring you such joy. In your life, you will hold a variety of opinions, many of which will evolve over time. However, don't feel obligated to hold them inside or to keep quiet because of your gender, external pressures, or fear. Whether it's in a journal or out loud, don't be hesitant to communicate your interests and opinions.

Embrace and accept your personal growth through puberty. This is how you hit back.

Hormone Imbalance

Teen females are known for being moody, private, and reluctant to discuss their developing bodies. Most often, people blame it on the fluctuating hormones of the adolescent years. How can you tell when your moods and physical changes have gone beyond what is normal and may point to a health problem?

Although teens' hormones are in transition, they can still become out of balance for a number of underlying reasons. A hormone imbalance can occasionally show in symptoms like delayed puberty or severe and rapid weight gain. In other instances, you might be unaware that you are showing signs of adolescent hormone imbalance, such as by having frequent menstrual periods. Because all of this is new to you, you might not recognize that something is wrong.

What Signs Indicate Teenage Hormone Imbalance?

Female teen hormone imbalance is frequently characterized by irregular or heavy periods, severe moodiness, exhaustion, weight gain, and facial hair. In addition, there are certain less common symptoms that, depending on the hormonal problems that a teen is experiencing, may appear in different combinations. Some of the signs include

- heightened sensitivity to heat or cold
- increased frequency of bowel movements or constipation
- dry skin
- round or puffy face
- unexplained weight gain or loss
- a higher or lower heart rate
- muscle trembling
- frequent urination
- increased thirst
- muscle or joint pain or stiffness
- loss of hair or thin, fragile hair
- increased appetite

- moodiness or worry
- distorted vision
- sweating
- an extra layer of fat between the shoulders
- stretch marks in purple or pink
- hot flashes
- craving for sugar
- fluid retention
- headache
- mental haze
- insomnia

What to Do if You Have Hormone Imbalances

Talk to your parents and have them take you to see your doctor. However, if you are experiencing only one or two of these symptoms, there's no need to panic or worry. Most times, it is just puberty being puberty. You may experience some of these signs but it doesn't necessarily mean you have a hormone imbalance.

Hence why it is crucial to talk to your parents about everything.

IS PUBERTY SCARY?

Puberty can be scary, especially if you don't have a female family member with whom you can talk about the changes and feelings you're experiencing. You can experience confusion or intense feelings that you've never experienced before during puberty. You can experience oversensitivity or have a quick temper, and this can sometimes be frightening.

You might also experience anxiety due to the way your body is changing.

Dealing with all these fresh feelings might be scary and hard at times, so it's crucial to understand that your mind is adjusting at the same time as your body to the new hormones. But the fear doesn't have to last long. Once you've grasped the idea that this is normal and your body will eventually be done going through these changes, you can move forward with loving yourself and giving your body, mind, and soul all the care they need through puberty.

Puberty is something that happens to all of us, so there is nothing to be ashamed of. Of course, fear can and might come, but the key is not to let it overpower you or rule the rest of your journey of growing up. Because, quite frankly, it's pretty awesome. You'll not only be introduced to the version of yourself that will be an adult someday, but the cool part is that you'll get more advantages of growing up. So, puberty is pretty awesome, and it can be our friend if we treat it right.

If you have a friend who you constantly reject, scorn, and feel ashamed of, do you think that friend will treat you kindly? The same goes for puberty. Treat yourself the way you want to be treated, and make the decision to refuse fear.

Another scary part of puberty is the fact that you can have sexual feelings that you have never had before, and you'll probably have a lot of questions concerning these strange, puzzling sexual feelings.

It's easy to feel awkward or uncomfortable when discussing sex, but, again, this is nothing to feel ashamed of. Remember those hormones called proges-terone and estrogen that we discussed earlier? I know a lot of girls won't like this part, but those very hormones are shaping your body to be sexually mature. Sexual feelings will come and you might find yourself feeling attracted to someone.

Try and get your doubts cleared, but make sure you have all the relevant facts first. Some children are able to discuss sex with their parents and receive all the information they need. But you can also talk to your doctor, a school counselor, a teacher, or any other adult you feel at ease talking to if you feel awkward discussing sex with your parents.

What you don't want to do is explore these feelings when you don't fully understand them. That can lead to hurt, heartbreak, and a whole lot of crying. Hold onto your innocence and the beauty of growing up. Always talk to a trusted adult about such feelings.

Yes, they can be scary, but they are just a part of your body's way of growing up.

BOYS CHANGE, TOO

Yes! It's not just girls who are experiencing these changes—boys are, too. You must have noticed boys who were once shorter than you suddenly tower over you, right? They have puberty to thank for that. Let's look at the changes that boys undergo when they get hit by puberty.

It's okay if you find this a bit weird, but it's important to note that this is normal and completely natural.

What Happens to Boys at Puberty

There are numerous signs that demonstrate that a boy is maturing during adolescence. Some of these include a growing body, changing voice, and new hair growth.

Puberty typically starts for boys between the ages of 9 and 14. However, puberty only begins when the body is prepared, and everyone develops at their own rate.

Height

A boy's height is influenced by his genes. It might depend on his mother, father, and other family members. However, nothing is certain. Some boys feel self-conscious about their height if they start puberty late, but exercises or magic drugs to increase height are not available. All he can do is eat healthily and wait for his time to shine.

Boys sometimes observe that girls reach adult height before they do. Girls typically begin these changes between the ages of 8 and 13, giving them a head start on puberty and growing taller. If you have a brother around your age, you might be taller than him for a few years. But watch out, he's coming right behind you.

Muscles

Some boys may have already begun to develop chest muscles. Some could have wide shoulders. However, there may still be some guys that are smaller and thinner.

Girls

Yep, girls are a part of boys' puberty just as they are a part of yours. Each boy has his own preferences. It's common for a boy to have crushes on people as he goes through puberty. If he doesn't right away, that's okay, too. Everyone is different.

Why do people have this feeling? With both boys and girls, it's all about the body's hormones becoming more active, so you begin to *feel* more as a result. These emotions may seem contradictory in boys and in girls. It's all in the process of transitioning into a new stage of life.

Body Hair

During puberty, body hair really begins to grow. For some guys, hair will start to appear above the lip, on the cheekbones, and around the chin. Additionally, hair grows on the chest, armpits, and even in the pubic area.

Because his body is receiving signals from hormones that it is ready to change, a boy develops hair in new areas. The adrenal glands produce some of the hormones that stimulate the growth of this new hair. They cause the testicles to enlarge and to begin secreting testosterone—a hormone that also encourages the growth of hair on the face, beneath the arms, and in the pubic region.

Body Odor

This is common in both boys and girls during puberty, and it might seem embarrassing, but it is a natural part of puberty. When your body becomes hot, sweat escapes from your skin through small openings known as pores.

Your hormones are constantly active during puberty. This is why you sweat frequently. With a few tiny quantities of additional substances, sweat is nearly entirely made up of water. By itself, sweat doesn't truly smell bad. However, it starts to smell when it comes into contact with skin bacteria that everyone has.

Teenagers may experience increased sweating and oily skin as their hormone levels rise during puberty. This is a typical stage of development, so it's crucial to cleanse your face every day. Acne might appear as a result of increased sweating as well.

Voice

As a boy grows, his voice becomes deeper. Their voice may occasionally "crack" during this period. This is a transitional occurrence that will stop over time.

Boys' Reproductive System in Puberty

Hormonal changes lead to the physical and sexual maturity that occurs throughout puberty.

It is challenging to predict the exact timing of puberty in boys. There are changes that take place, but they don't happen suddenly; they happen gradually over time. Boys go through particular stages of development as they acquire secondary sex traits.

Erections will start to occur in boys (this is when a boy's penis fills with blood and becomes hard). Erections might occur for no apparent reason or when they think about sexual matters. Boys may also have something known as nocturnal emissions, or wet dreams.

The body of a boy starts producing sperm throughout puberty. During an erection, semen, which is composed of sperm and other bodily fluids, may be released. The term for this is ejaculation. Because of the possibility that his underwear or the bed may be somewhat wet when he wakes up, these are known as "wet dreams." As boys progress through adolescence, wet dreams become less frequent and eventually end. This is a normal aspect of adolescence. With this change, a boy now has the possibility of getting someone pregnant.

For boys, hormones pass through the bloodstream and instruct the testes (the sac that hangs below the penis) to start producing testosterone and sperm. The majority of the physical changes that occur in a boy's body throughout puberty are brought on by the hormone testosterone.

STAGES OF PUBERTY

Teenagers go through a lot of changes during puberty which eventually comes to an end when the body has fully matured. Teenagers may find the various stages hard or even confusing, especially given that each person experiences these changes at a different pace.

The "Tanner stages" explain how the body alters and the symptoms to look out for at each stage.

What Are the Tanner Stages of Puberty?

The first person to recognize the outward signs of puberty was child development specialist Professor James M. Tanner (Marcin, 2022).

These phases are now referred to as the Tanner stages or, more accurately, sexual maturity ratings (SMRs). Despite the fact that every person experiences puberty at a different time, they serve as a basic guide to physical growth.

The Tanner stages also describe the stages of female puberty and when they are most likely to take place.

They are a great resource for anticipating the changes you will go through. For girls, there are five stages of puberty.

Stage One—Brain Signals

Tanner stage one highlights your development before any outward signs of puberty show. It normally begins after you turn eight. These internal modifications are the same in both males and females.

- The body starts receiving signals from the brain to adjust to the changes.
- Gonadotropin-releasing hormone (GnRH), which the pituitary gland uses to produce hormones that regulate other glands in the body, starts to be released by the brain.
- Luteinizing hormone (LH) and follicle-stimulating hormone (FSH) are two more hormones that the pituitary gland begins to produce.
- At this point, you may not perceive any physical changes.

Stage Two—Physical Development

Stage two marks the start of bodily changes. This is when your body starts to receive signals from hormones. Typically, girls between the ages of 8 and 13 go through the following changes:

- Under the nipple, the "buds" that will eventually become breasts begin to appear. One bud could be larger than the other, which is normal, and they may be painful or tender to the touch.
- The darker area (areola) surrounding the nipple will enlarge.
- Small portions of pubic hair start to sprout, and the uterus starts to expand.
- Every year, height increases by around two-and-a-half inches.

Stage Three—Growth Spurts and More

In stage three, your physical changes become more pronounced. Your hormones are hard at work causing a growth spurt in height and advancing development from the earlier stages.

Females typically experience physical changes around and beyond the age of 12. These adjustments include:

- Breast "buds" are still developing and enlarging.
- Pubic hair thickens and becomes curlier. Pubic hair grows in a triangular shape and is coarse and curly.

- The armpits begin to grow hair.
- Acne forms as skin becomes oilier. Acne may first appear on the back and face.
- The fastest growth rates for height start (around 3.2 inches per year).
- Fat begins to accumulate on the hips and thighs.

Stage Four—Puberty in Full Swing

In stage four, puberty reaches its peak. These changes happen between 13 and 15 years old:

- Nipples begin to protrude as they move past the bud stage, and your breasts continue to develop and take on a fuller shape.
- There are now far too many pubic hairs to count, but they are still arranged in a triangle.
- The rate of growth in height will decrease to 2 to 3 inches annually.
- Acne problems can persist.
- Most females experience their first period between the ages of 12 and 14, though it can occur earlier or later.

Stage Five—Entering Adolescence

The conclusion of your growth starts with stage five. You will finally reach your full physical development during this last stage, including your full adult height.

In this stage, development usually comes to an end. Girls grow physically into adults. Although most girls reach their maximum height by the age of 16, some may continue to grow until they are 20. Stage five often begins in females around the age of 15. Changes include the following:

- The size and shape of the breasts resemble those of an adult, though they can still change up until the age of 18.
- After a few years, periods start to become regular.
- One to two years following their first period, females reach adult height.
- Inner thighs are covered in pubic hair.
- Reproductive organs are fully formed.
- The form of buttocks, thighs, and hips is improved.

Puberty does not occur suddenly. Numerous physical and hormonal changes occur over the course of many years, and they can all be difficult to go through.

You are probably feeling a lot right now, whether it be about menstruation, acne, body odor, or something else. While expressing these feelings, be open with your parents or guardian. You will need someone to support you in this stage of your development. What you are experiencing is normal and part of puberty, and it doesn't have to be a terrible period of your development.

Everyone goes through puberty at their own rate. It's possible that you haven't yet developed breasts while a few of your friends are starting their periods. Perhaps your best friend's body has changed, but you still believe you look young. Or perhaps it's the other way around, and you're tired of being the tallest girl in your class.

Kids who enter puberty extremely late or who develop very quickly can have issues that may need to be examined or treated. If that prospect worries you, talk to your parents and make an appointment with your doctor. Your doctor can assess if you are developing appropriately because they are experts on puberty.

However, most people catch up eventually, and the majority of the differences between you and your peers will disappear. Hold on till that time comes. The teenage years can be pretty exciting!

PERIOD PENNINGS

Let's reflect!

Take a few minutes to reflect on your journey through puberty so far, or what you expect in the years to come. You can start like this:

1. So far, the changes I've noticed in my body are…
2. What I love about puberty is…
3. What I dislike about puberty is…
4. Do you find puberty scary? If yes, what can you do to embrace and take control of this moment of life? If no, what can you share with your friends and family going through the same thing?

_____
_____
_____
_____
_____
_____
_____
_____
_____
_____
_____
_____

Segue: The next chapter talks about the changes that girls experience during this time.

CHANGES IN YOUR BODY

re you afraid of the pimples and acne on your face? Do you feel uncomfortable in your clothes because you keep outgrowing them? Do you feel like you need a bra, slip, or something else to cover your chest properly? We might've touched on a few of these topics in previous chapters, but here we'll talk in more detail about these changes.

Let's understand these changes a bit better. Buckle up, because this is going to be a fun ride!

VISIBLE CHANGES IN YOUR BODY

As we all know, young teens go through a lot of physical changes when they enter puberty, including changes in size and shape, development of pubic and underarm hair, and an increase in body odor. Breast growth and the beginning of menstruation are two examples of changes that affect us as girls.

In classes and among peers, this is the time when your physical traits change the most; some may develop to the point that, by the end of the school term, you may be too big for the desks you were given at the start of the school year! On the other hand, others might develop slower.

Early adolescence frequently comes with fresh worries about looks and body image. Girls and boys who previously didn't give their appearance a second thought may suddenly spend hours primping, fretting, and fussing about being too little, too tall, too chubby, too slim, or too pimply. Different body parts may develop at varying rates. For instance, hands and feet may develop more quickly than arms and legs. You may be clumsy and uncomfortable in your physical activities because moving your body requires a partnership of all bodily components, and these parts are changing sizes.

The pace of a young teen's physical growth and development can also have an impact on other areas of their life. A girl who reaches puberty at the age of 11 will have different interests from a girl who does not until she is 14. Young adolescents who mature very early or really late may face particular issues.

Late bloomers may believe they can't take part in sports with their classmates who are more physically developed. Conversely, those who mature more quickly could be forced into adult roles before they're emotionally or mentally prepared for them.

Long-lasting impacts may result from the link between the age at which physical changes associated with puberty begin and how friends, classmates, family, and the environment around them react to those changes.

However, some preteens relish the notion that they are maturing independently of their friends. For instance, they might have an edge over peers who mature later, particularly in athletics.

Many young teens, regardless of their rate of growth, have unrealistic views of who they are, and they require reassurance that everyone grows at a different rate. In this section, we'll discuss some of these physical changes, what happens, and how you can embrace and control them. Knowing that they are natural and normal, you should love yourself regardless of your rate of growth or that of those around you.

What Is Acne?

Acne is a common skin problem in which hair, sebum (an oily fluid), germs, and dead skin cells clog the pores of your skin. Blackheads, whiteheads, pimples, and cysts are some of the numerous forms of bumps that appear as acne. The hormone changes associated with puberty are the cause of acne in teenagers. You have a higher likelihood of getting acne if your parents did when they were teenagers. However, by the time most people are out of their teens, their acne has virtually vanished.

The most common areas of the body where acne appears on the skin are the face, chest, shoulders, and upper back. Teenagers are frequently affected by acne, but it can affect anyone. Due to its prevalence, acne is considered a typical aspect of puberty.

Know that you are not alone if you have acne. The majority of people encounter this skin issue. According to estimates, 80% of individuals between the ages of 11 and 30 will experience acne of some kind at some point in their life (*Acne*, 2020).

Puberty Pimples

It's a well-known fact that preteens and teenagers experience changes. Acne can occasionally be the outcome of those changes. This section is for you if you're one of the numerous adolescents who experience acne during puberty! Let's discuss the factors that contribute to teen acne, how to prevent it from developing, and what to do if pimples do appear.

Types of Acne

There are various types of acne. They consist of the following:

- **Blackheads**: These are open skin lumps that collect extra oil and dead skin. The black patches, which mimic dirt deposits, are actually generated by an uneven light reflection off the blocked pore.
- **Whiteheads**: These are bumpy areas that are kept closed by skin debris and oil.
- **Papules**: Tiny pimples that are red or pink and swell up.
- **Pustules**: These are pus-filled pimples. They have the appearance of red rings encircling whiteheads. If they are picked or scratched, they may leave scars.
- **Pityrosporum folliculitis** (fungal acne): This is brought on by an overgrowth of yeast in the hair follicles. They can become swollen and itchy.

- **Nodules**: Firm zits buried deep beneath the skin. They are large and can be painful.
- **Cysts**: Acne that is pus-filled. These might leave scars.

Your self-esteem may be impacted by any of these acne types. It is advisable to consult your healthcare professional as soon as possible so that they can assist you in choosing the appropriate treatment option(s).

Causes of Acne

Puberty is the primary cause of acne in teenagers, though there are other causes as well. Your hormone levels are changing which may cause your skin's pores and hair follicles to produce more oil. Your pores may become clogged by this extra oil, dead skin cells, and bacteria, which can result in acne.

Additionally, acne can run in families; if one or both of your parents struggled with acne as adolescents, chances are that you will as well. Another typical cause of acne in preteens and teenagers is stress.

Acne can also be brought on by these factors:

- hormone levels that change around your period
- picking at an acne scar
- wearables like hats, sports helmets, and clothing

- pollution in the air and specific weather conditions, particularly excessive humidity
- using oily personal care products such as thick creams, lotions, or waxes, or being in an environment where you frequently come into contact with grease
- increased cortisol levels that cause stress
- some medicines

Androgen hormones, which normally become active during adolescence and young adulthood, are also a major hormonal factor in acne. Acne can be brought on by sensitivity to these hormones in addition to surface skin bacteria and fatty acids within oil glands. During the teen years, certain hormones reach their highest levels.

How Can You Prevent Acne?

Preventing acne from developing in the first place is the best method to treat it. Even if it's impossible to prevent pimples from appearing because it is caused by puberty, the following helpful habits should greatly benefit your skin:

- Once or twice a day, wash your face with warm water and mild soap or cleanser. Scrubbing your face vigorously with a washcloth won't get rid of acne and could make it more severe by irritating your skin and pores. Make an effort to wash your face as tenderly and gently as you can.

- Wash your face after working out or doing any form of high physical activity to remove sweat from your pores.

- To reduce inflammation and the transmission of bacteria from your hands, avoid touching your hands to your face or picking at your skin or current acne.

- Keep hair gels and sprays away from your face if you use them because they can potentially block pores. Wash your hair regularly to remove oil if you have long hair that touches your face.

- If you frequently get acne on your forehead, keep your hair off your face and stay away from low-brim hats.

- There are numerous over-the-counter products that contain benzoyl peroxide or salicylic acid that can both prevent acne and treat it. Try several combinations to find which works best for you. Don't use more of the product than is recommended to avoid overdrying your skin and making it feel and look worse. Also, pay attention to any warnings on the label regarding allergies.

- Use a moisturizer recommended by your doctor or dermatologist.
- Some individuals discover that eating an excessive amount of a particular food causes their breakouts to worsen. If you fall into this category, you should try reducing your intake of that type of food to see what happens.

Here's another point that I wanted to emphasize: Do not touch, pinch, or pick at a pimple that you see. It can be very tempting to try to get rid of a pimple, so this might be challenging. However, if you play with pimples, popping or opening them up will worsen the inflammation that is already there. Additionally, the oils on your hands can worsen it. Furthermore, picking at pimples can result in tiny scars on your face.

Can scars from acne appear?

The answer is yes. Scarring from acne does occur occasionally.

It occurs when acne destroys the deeper layers of the skin by invading them. Inflammation causes the pore walls to break down, causing the acne pores to swell.

Of course, scarring can cause anxiety, which is normal. Still, we want to prevent it as much as possible, right? Perhaps there will be a little scarring either way, but you can do your part by refusing to pick at your skin.

Your future self will thank you for it.

Skin Care Tips for Acne

Let's have a little fun experimenting with finding a self-care routine that works for you. As you grow older, you'll find yourself more and more enticed by self-care routines, which are wonderful things for us to do.

When you're in your adolescence and your body is already starting to change rapidly, you should start practicing good skin care. It can assist you in maintaining healthy skin and preventing premature aging from posing concerns in the future.

Many girls start with a skin care routine in their adolescence, usually to either treat pimples or maintain their glow—or both. So I've compiled a list of skin care tips that you can add to your morning and nightly routines.

Do not try all of these tips at once; instead, see which ones you are most comfortable with and what works best for you. What works for me won't necessarily work for you, but there is something here for you, I'm sure.

You only need the appropriate products for your skin type, the appropriate methods, and the determination to take care of your skin every day.

1. Use a mild cleanser

Use a cleanser made for your skin type when washing your face correctly to prevent irritating or drying out your skin. Avoid vigorous scrubbing; instead, use soft circular strokes to thoroughly clean your face.

You can also reduce the amount of sebum (oil) produced and the prevalence of blackheads by taking vitamin A or zinc supplements.

2. Drink plenty of water

Drinking water will keep your skin bright and hydrated. Drink a glass of water to start your day. When you go to school, have a bottle of water with you. Drink from it throughout the day.

If drinking water sounds uninteresting and bland, give it a twist by adding slices of lemons, cucumbers, star fruit, or grapefruit. You can try any of these and see which you prefer.

3. Weekly exfoliation

Keep your skin exfoliated (which means removing dead skin) to prevent clogged pores brought on by hormonal changes.

Alpha hydroxy acids (AHA) and salicylic acid-based chemical exfoliators are excellent methods for cleaning deeply into your pores. It's okay if you have no clue what these are. Ask your parents or someone older to accompany you when you go shopping for products! It can be fun.

4. Moisturize regularly

Use moisturizer twice a day to keep your skin hydrated and smooth and to delay the appearance of wrinkles and lines. If you have oily skin, be sure to apply a mild, oil-free moisturizer to avoid clogging. If your face is prone to acne, you can also use moisturizers with a gel base.

To help shield your skin from the sun's rays, you might select a moisturizer that also functions as a broad-spectrum sunscreen. Avoid using moisturizers with extra fragrance if you have delicate skin.

5. Maintain a balanced diet

Consume a diet rich in fruits and vegetables for balance. Eat less sugary and fatty food because they can make your skin conditions worse.

Avoid dairy products like cow's milk if you can. You can pick plant-based milk like oat milk or almond milk as a substitute. Look for foods high in healthy fats, such as salmon, avocados, and almonds.

6. Commit to a good nighttime skincare routine

While you're sleeping, your skin renews itself. Before going to bed, be sure to wash your face, erase all dirt and cosmetics, and then moisturize.

7. Choose a healthy lifestyle

Take control of your body as a young person. The general health of your body immediately affects the condition of your skin. Exercise, meditation practices, a nutritious diet, and drinking lots of water are all recommended.

8. Use lukewarm water

Always wash your face twice daily with warm (not scorching hot) water. It aids in removing the debris while preserving the naturally moisturizing oils in your skin.

9. Take care of your lips

Your lips require care just the same as your facial skin does! Before heading to bed, use lip balm. You can cleanse your lips as well. Wet your lips, put a little cream on a baby toothbrush, scrub gently for one minute, and finish with lip balm. It'll feel smooth and soft.

10. Consult with a doctor

A dermatologist visit can make a significant difference, particularly if you have painful, big lumps under the skin or red, pus-filled pimples. Prescription washes and acne medications, which can clear skin more quickly and efficiently than over-the-counter items, may be beneficial to you.

Creating a skincare routine is important, but sticking to it consistently is even more important! You may lose patience and expect immediate results, but keep in mind that skincare is a process and an adventure!

Maintain a single regimen and give it time to produce benefits. Continue to use the products you are currently using if they are appropriate for your skin type. Try not to change your routine or products too much past the initial stage of experimenting.

What Are Breast Buds

As we know, girls often start going through puberty between the ages of 8 and 13. For the majority of girls, the appearance of coin-sized bumps underneath the nipple, known as breast "buds," is the first sign of puberty. Breast growth frequently begins in one breast before the other.

With breast buds, you might experience some tenderness or pain, but soreness and uneven breast growth are completely natural and usually resolve themselves over time. You may experience both excitement and fear as you adjust to your changing body during this time. It's sometimes a bittersweet experience when breasts start to bud.

What Takes Place While the Breasts Develop?

Breast buds, which appear in the initial stage of what is known as breast development, are characterized by a tiny swelling under the nipple.

Your breasts may be extremely sensitive and painful when they first begin to develop. As your skin stretches, they might also itch. A bra can help protect developing breasts and lessen discomfort. Stretch marks may develop on the skin if the breasts expand quickly. Over time, these will disappear.

As a girl reaches puberty, her body fat increases, and the breasts continue to develop. They expand and round out. The nipple might be erect or stick out, and the areola (the region surrounding the nipple) may become darker and bigger.

One breast frequently develops more quickly than the other. Although it should eventually balance out, many adult women discover that their breasts are very slightly different in size. Don't worry, this is entirely normal.

Will My Breasts Grow in Size?

Genetics plays a major role in determining your breast size. Girls' breast sizes will increase with weight gain since breasts contain fat cells. You have no control over how quickly or slowly breast development occurs. However, it's important that we understand that breast sizes will be different for everyone, so love your breasts and the size they are. Comparing your breast size to others' will do more harm than good.

It's natural to wonder if your breasts are normal. However, everyone's breasts are unique and come in a variety of shapes and sizes.

Changes During Menstruation

Your breasts may change throughout your monthly cycle due to hormonal changes. Swelling, discomfort, and sensitivity may be among these monthly changes, and in certain circumstances, the texture of the breasts may change, making them feel lumpier.

Growing Taller

Girls experience rapid growth in birth and childhood, but when you hit adolescence, your rate of development increases once more. In general, girls experience a significant growth spurt between the ages of 10 and 14. One to two years before the beginning of menstruation is when girls often experience a growth spurt. By the time you are 14 or 15 years old, or a few years after menstruation begins, you might stop growing and attain your adult height. In the year or two following the start of your first period, you will probably only gain one to two more inches in height.

Quick facts about girls' growth:

- Puberty typically begins and ends for females before it does for males.
- Everyone enters puberty at a different age, even though there is a common age range for when it begins.
- Around age 11 or 12, females often experience their fastest growth spurt.

Other factors that may affect height include:

- **Nutrition**: Children who are undernourished are frequently smaller and shorter than average for their age. However, kids might be capable of catching up before adulthood with a good diet.
- **Hormonal imbalances**: For instance, low growth hormone levels might cause delayed growth and shorter adult heights.
- **Medications**: Some medications have the potential to slow growth.
- **Chronic disease**: Long-term health issues like cystic fibrosis, kidney illness, and celiac disease might cause a height that is lower than average.

- **Genetics**: There are many variations in "normal" height since genetics play a big role in determining growth patterns. The heights of your parents have a significant impact on your own height. Growth traits tend to run in families.

Through adolescence, you may grow a whole foot taller! Or you may not. But, like everything else in puberty, it is different for everyone, so you might not be as tall as some people or as short as others.

You can develop in a healthy way with the support of excellent habits like getting adequate sleep, eating wholesome foods, and exercising frequently.

Stretch Marks

Stretch marks are just as common in teenagers as in adults, if not more so. Stretch marks can appear on a teenager's legs, shoulders, belly, chest, and other locations due to the significant physical changes brought on by puberty.

Stretch marks are tiny lines on the skin that appear as a result of rapid weight gain or growth (like during puberty). Although skin is typically quite elastic, excessive stretching can cause a disruption in the regular creation of collagen, which is a significant protein that contributes to the structure of skin tissue. As a result, stretch marks may appear.

Stretch marks first may appear as reddish or purplish lines that may resemble dents and have a different texture than the surrounding skin.

These stretch marks are not harmful, though, and can be decreased with both natural cures and professional care. Eventually, they might disappear on their own as well. In this section, we will cover every aspect of teenage stretch marks and how to treat them. So, if you have noticed stretch marks on your body, this part is for you.

What Do They Look Like?

The appearance of your stretch marks can vary depending on a number of factors including

- your skin's natural color
- the condition and elasticity of your skin
- the impacted body part

In general, these lines are not the same color or texture as the rest of your skin. They can be purple, crimson, light gray, or pale in color. Stretch mark warning signs and symptoms include

- indented lines or streaks that can vary in size and length (depending on the color of your skin)
- pink, purple, red, bluish, or dark brown color
- thin, glossy lines in your skin that may turn whitish over time
- skin itchiness and irritation before stretch marks develop

Stretch Marks in Teens: Are They Normal?

Stretch marks appearing on teenagers is, in fact, very normal. Teenagers may go through a dramatic growth spurt around this time, and stretch marks may appear on some portions of their bodies. Stretch marks typically appear in these places on teenagers:

- hips
- buttocks
- thighs
- breasts
- abdomen
- upper back and lower back (including the shoulders)
- upper arms
- legs and knees

Do Stretch Marks Go Away?

Over time, stretch marks may develop in new places and those that already exist may gradually disappear. However, if you want to take matters into your own hands, there are some things that you may do to help get rid of stretch marks.

Stretch marks can be reduced in size or perhaps totally eliminated with the use of many treatments and methods. Still, they might not always be effective or provide benefits right away. Here are a few of those treatments:

- **Moisturizer**. There are many moisturizers that help with the reduction or removal of stretch marks. If you want to try one, massage it gently into fresh stretch marks over a period of a few weeks.
- **Lotion for self-tanner**. Using a self-tanner might temporarily reduce the difference between the color of your regular skin tone and the color of your stretch marks.
- **Prescription creams**. Several prescription skin treatments may help early stretch marks become less visible. These include tretinoin, a synthetic form of vitamin A, and hyaluronic acid. You may ask your parents or doctor to help you choose the right one.

Although you might find stretch marks to be unpleasant, they are normal and often temporary, and there are no long-term health problems associated with stretch marks.

So, if you do develop stretch marks and your first reaction is dislike, that's okay. But you can also learn to accept and embrace them because you are not alone and they are just another indicator that you are growing up to be a beautiful young woman. Until they fade (if they fade), let them shine and love them as you would love anything else about your body.

Cellulite

The lumpy skin texture that is frequently seen on the butt, stomach, and thighs is known as cellulite. The connective tissue that lies beneath the skin is pushed apart by fat, giving the skin's surface a bumpy appearance. Before we go any farther with this section, I think it's crucial to highlight that cellulite is completely natural, common, and acceptable.

Cellulite is quite normal and having a few lumps and bumps on your body doesn't make it "disgusting" or "ruined." It's actually not a huge deal at all. Pinching the skin on your upper thigh will reveal whether you have cellulite. You might have it if the area you pinched appears a little lumpy. You are most definitely not alone if you do have cellulite. Cellulite is common among women and girls.

Cellulite is influenced by a number of factors, including

- **Genes**. Typically, cellulite runs in families.
- **Gender**. Girls and women are more likely than boys and men to have cellulite.
- **Weight**. Cellulite can exist in thin people, but it's more visible in those with higher body fat percentages.
- **Age**. With age, cellulite becomes more prevalent.

It cannot be cured by any miracle creams, therapies, or medications. Some "treatments" might momentarily make cellulite appear less noticeable. Though cellulite typically appears after puberty, if you ever discover cellulite, keep a healthy weight and engage in an exercise routine. Cellulite will be less noticeable if you replace fat with muscle.

Though it has been brushed under the carpet as if it's something ugly, it happens to every woman and it is nothing to be ashamed of. These are your genes—own them, girl!

Body Hair

This might be one of your least favorite aspects of puberty, but you'll start to notice your hair thickening or growing in new places. You will develop hair in your pubic region—which is close to your vagina—on your legs, and in your armpits. As you get older, this hair will start off thin and straight and then thicken and occasionally get curlier.

Why Do We Have Body Hair?

On average, there are five million hair follicles on our bodies, from the scalp to the pubic region to our toes (Kinonen, 2020).

While you might not grow additional hair as you get older, the amount and distribution of the hair you do have changes over time. Depending on where it is located on your body, your hair matures and changes as you age.

For instance, the hair on your head, pubic region, and underarms is referred to as terminal hair and is visibly thicker and stronger than the rest of the body's hair. Vellus hair is the softer, thinner hair that covers the majority of the remainder of your body. However, as you age, vellus hair might change into terminal hair due to hormones.

The reasons we have hair in particular places on our bodies, however, are actually pretty fascinating. For instance, the primary function of the hair on our heads is to control the temperature of our brains.

You've probably noticed that in addition to the hair on our heads, it also grows thickly in a few other areas of the body, like the armpits, the pubic area, and the brows. Hair in the pubic area and underarms is important because it distributes odor molecules. Even though we occasionally try to get rid of odor molecules, some of them are crucial for communicating things like our reproductive status.

Compared to underarm or pubic hair, eyebrows serve a completely different function. Even from a distance, people may be able to tell what our expressions and moods are by looking at our brows. Additionally, eyebrows protect our eyes from sweat.

But what about the hair that isn't as visible on the body? Just be aware that it is still present and serves an important purpose. Our body is covered in incredibly tiny hairs that are crucial for us because they enable our skin to heal properly. They are tiny stem cell vaults that aid in the healing of our wounds. The hair on our skin also helps to control our body temperature; when we are cold, the hair on our body sticks out, acting as a protective shield from the cold, and when we are hot, the hair on our body lays flat to allow air to pass over our skin and cool us down.

The red of your lips, your palms, and the soles of your feet are the only parts of your body that don't have hair while the remainder of your skin is covered in these little hairs.

We don't have hair on our lips since they are made up of a different sort of cell than the rest of our bodies. Cool, isn't it?

Body Hair Removal

This is what we know so far: Each hair follicle performs a number of essential tasks in the overall operation of the human body. So, why have we been removing hair from certain parts of our bodies for the past few centuries? You can credit that to social and cultural traditions and norms, I suppose.

Of course, if you decide to get rid of your body hair—which is totally fine!—there are a variety of techniques you can use depending on where the hair is located.

Shaving

The first option is shaving, which involves using a razor to remove hair. You remove hair from above the top layer of skin when you shave your body (usually on the legs, underarms, bikini area, and face). To keep the skin hydrated, shaving with a cream or gel is advised.

- **How it works**: You cut off the hair shaft's tip that has grown through the skin with a razor. Some razors have a replaceable blade, some are electronic, and some are fully disposable.
- **Longevity**: It lasts for one to three days.
- **Advantages**: You can do it yourself and shaving is not too expensive. All you need is some warm water, a blade, and shaving cream or gel if you desire.
- **Disadvantages**: Shaving can cause razor burns, bumps, scratches, cuts, and ingrown hairs. Ingrown hairs occur when the hair starts to grow and it does not emerge from the follicle but rather develops underneath the surrounding tissue. The skin becomes irritated when the hair begins to curl and grow into it. Ingrown hairs can be avoided by shaving in the direction that the hair develops, despite the fact that most individuals do the reverse.
- **Tips**: Shave in the shower when your skin has already been moistened by warm water for a better shave. When using the razor on looser skin, be gentle and go slowly. To prevent cuts, change razors frequently. Protecting delicate

skin, such as the skin surrounding the genitals, may also be aided by using shaving cream. Try using an electric razor if you're afraid of cutting yourself.

Tweezing

Unlike shaving, tweezing removes the hair right from the follicle. You might imagine a hair follicle as the tiny home where your hair lives. A hair will always grow back after being pulled out of a follicle. However, it will take more time than if you merely remove it from the above skin as with shaving.

- **How it works**: Tightly stretch the skin and hold the hair by the root and pull it out with tweezers.
- **Longevity**: It lasts for three to eight weeks.
- **Advantages**: It is cost-effective as all you require are tweezers. However, because you are only able to pluck one hair at a time, it can take some time.
- **Disadvantages**: Tweezing might be painful. An ingrown hair can occur if the hair splits off beneath the skin. You could get temporary red bumps after plucking since the hair follicle is inflamed and swollen.

- **Tips**: To lessen the risk of infection, make sure to clean your tweezers or other plucking tools with rubbing alcohol before and after use.

Waxing

Similar to tweezing, waxing pulls hair out of the follicle by placing the warm wax on the skin's surface and around the hair. You basically yank the hair from the follicle when you remove the wax.

- **How it works**: On the skin area where the hair is growing, apply a sticky wax. The hair roots and dead skin are then removed by applying a cloth strip over the wax and quickly peeling it off. Both at home and in a salon are options for waxing.
- **Longevity**: It lasts for three to six weeks.
- **Advantages**: Waxing makes the skin smooth and lasts a long time. It's easy to find waxing kits in pharmacies and supermarkets. Compared to other hair removal treatments like shaving, hair regrowth after waxing seems lighter and less obvious.
- **Disadvantages**: According to many, pain and soreness are the main negative sides to waxing. The removal of the hair can hurt a little because the treatment pulls hair out from the roots, but

fortunately, that process only takes a few minutes. Following waxing, some people may experience brief redness, irritation, or pimples.

- **Tips**: Hair should be at least 1/4 inch (about 6 millimeters) long for waxing to be effective, so go a few weeks before you wax without shaving. Waxing shouldn't be done on moles or sunburned skin.

The cost of professional waxing is higher than that of other hair removal techniques. Although there is no need to be ashamed, it might be beneficial to have your first waxing procedure done at a salon so you can observe how the experts do it. Salon workers are trained to wax all areas of the male and female bodies.

Depilatory Cream

In this method, you apply a chemical that dissolves the hair at the root rather than grasping and pulling at it, and you essentially just wipe it away. It functions by reacting with the hair's protein structure, causing the hair to break down.

While effective at removing hair, depilatory lotions have some additional risks. You may experience severe skin irritability if some of the chemicals enter the follicle, which they often do. This is because the chemicals impact your follicles.

- **How they work**: Follow the directions on the packaging and apply depilatory cream to the desired area. Remove by washing or wiping the cream away.
- **Longevity**: They last for a few days to two weeks.
- **Advantages**: Depilatories are affordable, easily accessible at pharmacies and grocery stores, and they work swiftly. They work well on the legs, underarms, and bikini area.
- **Disadvantages**: Depilatories can be messy to apply, and many individuals find the smell unpleasant. If you have delicate skin, you may experience an allergic reaction to the depilatory's ingredients, which could result in a rash or irritation. Depilatory creams might not work as well on coarse hair.
- **Tips**: For optimal results, follow the product recommendations carefully and make sure you use the product as directed. Read product labels to identify a depilatory that is approved for use on the "bikini area" before applying it to pubic hair.

Laser Removal

Lasers don't work on light hair since they target the pigmentation in the hair follicle.

- **How it works**: A laser is used to halt the growth of hair by passing through the skin and into the hair follicle. Since the melanin (colored pigment) in dark hair absorbs more light, it is most effective on those with light skin and dark hair.
- **Longevity**: Although it might be permanent, maintenance calls for regular visits every six to twelve months.
- **Advantages**: Large areas of skin can be treated simultaneously, and this method of hair removal is long-lasting.
- **Disadvantages**: Sessions can cost up to $400. Redness and inflammation are potential treatment side effects.
- **Tips**: Applying cold compresses after the treatment may help reduce inflammation. Prior to receiving the procedure, avoiding the sun may improve results.

Exfoliate both before and after treatment—regardless of the hair removal method you select—to give the hair the best chance of penetrating beneath the skin's surface and emerging from it. Ingrown hairs could result from not doing this. Ingrown hairs are fairly common, but if they're not treated, they can become very unpleasant and even infected.

Still, ensure you do thorough research on whatever method of removal you choose, and always have a parent or guardian supervising you for the first couple of times until you really get the hang of it (no matter how embarrassing it might seem). You should also do patch tests (trying the method on a small section of your arm or leg before doing the entire area) to find what works best for you. Talk to your mom or a trusted adult to help you, and avoid following social media trends for hair removal.

Body hair is an essential, natural element in the human structure. Your body hair and what you do with it are completely up to you. You can either choose to accept it or get rid of it.

The decision to remove body hair is a personal one. Nobody is healthier if they have less body hair, so you shouldn't feel compelled to get rid of it if you don't want to. Do what seems appropriate to you, and most importantly, continue loving yourself through it all!

OKAY, ONE MORE THING...

Some teenagers feel that they are too thin and question if they should make changes. While gaining weight during adolescence is common, aiming to do so might not be the best course of action.

Does Puberty Make You Fat?

During puberty, your body grows and changes shape.

Typically, the bodies of girls get curvier. As we know, your nipples initially swell somewhat, and then your hips become broader and your breasts begin to form.

Some girls may feel uncomfortable with how their figures are changing due to all the growing and developing they are doing, but dieting to prevent any typical weight gain is unhealthy. Speak to your parents, doctor, or school counselor if you have any concerns about your weight or puberty.

On the other hand, some girls might feel compelled to do more to gain weight. This, too, should be avoided.

Whatever your motivation for wanting to put on weight may be, the majority of teenagers have no need to do so. Your risk for health issues may grow as you gain more weight, so prioritize your health and strength instead of your weight. One of your responsibilities as a teen is to maintain physical fitness so that your body can develop properly.

Here are some actions you can take to accomplish this:

- Set nutrition as a priority. Healthy eating doesn't have to be difficult. Eating a range of healthy foods can benefit your body more than trying to gain weight by consuming unhealthy foods.
- Make time to eat meals and snacks on a regular basis and consume a range of healthful foods. Never eat past the point of feeling full.
- Frequently eat fruits and vegetables.
- Eat whole grains.
- Eat breakfast daily.
- Eat nutritious snacks.
- Limit unhealthy choices like soda and chips.

At this stage of your life, eating healthily is crucial for a variety of reasons. Normal growth is dependent upon proper nourishment and exercise. Good eating habits can be developed now and will eventually become automatic. Without you realizing it, this will assist you in maintaining your physical health.

PERIOD PENNINGS

Let's reflect!

Think about everything you've learned in this chapter. Are there any changes in your physique that you have noticed? Write them down! Here are a few questions that can help with your journaling:

1. If there is one thing I could do right now without any restrictions, it would be...
2. Physical changes make me anxious because...
3. I like/dislike the changes in my body because...
4. What can I do to always accept and embrace the changes in my body?
5. Do you have acne? If yes, what skin care technique would you like to try?

_____
_____
_____
_____
_____
_____
_____
_____
_____
_____

Segue: The next chapter talks about starting your period for the first time.

STARTING YOUR PERIOD

N ow here comes the peak of female puberty development—the only thing from puberty that will stay with us for decades.

Our period.

As discussed in the previous chapters, the changes in the body that you observe act as the first signs that your period is coming. When you start to notice these changes in your body, be extra aware because you never know when the bell of your period will actually ring; being prepared is better unless you want your first period story to be mortifying. Speaking of mortifying stories, check this one out:

In the sixth grade, we prepared for days for the spelling bee contest. I had been noticing a few changes in my body, but I was too focused on the contest to give them much thought. Of course, you can imagine what happened next.

I stood behind the pulpit, spitting out words of fire like the last dragon, when my opponent tugged on my shirt and showed me a blotch of red on the back of my pants. I was mortified, of course, but I knew it was my period from all the stories my mom had told me. However, at that moment, it didn't occur to me that I could just spell a word wrong so I could leave the contest. No, I stuck out to the end, spelling word after word in front of the entire school for the next hour.

I won the contest with the word "pneumonia," by the way, but I was—and still am—haunted by that moment.

This doesn't have to be you, or maybe it has been you. That's the funny thing with periods. Every month it's a spelling bee contest hazard all over again, and that's just the reality for us girls. In the end, although you can be extra prepared, it is still an unpredictable situation, and if you get caught in the crosshairs of it, don't be too hard on yourself. It's okay. It happens to everyone.

WHEN WILL I GET MY FIRST PERIOD?

A young woman's first period marks a significant turning point in her life. It marks the start of a lengthy period of time (about 40 years!) during which you may be fertile. This means that you could become pregnant if you have sexual intercourse. Even if you studied menstruation in school, you probably still have concerns about what to expect. This section is intended to provide you with all the knowledge you require as you approach having your first period.

About two years after your breasts first begin to form is when your period will likely appear. When blood is shed through the vagina, it is known as the menstrual period. That may sound concerning, but it's natural and shows that a girl is maturing and her body is getting ready for the possibility of having a child in the future.

What Causes Menstruation?

Puberty leads to the start of menstruation, at which point your body can start reproducing.

Your estrogen levels rise when your menstrual cycle starts, and your uterus's lining thickens as a result.

Your body will loosen and shed the lining and push it from your uterus if there isn't a fertilized egg. This specific kind of bleeding is your menstrual period.

Periods can be challenging to manage regardless of how long you have had them or whether this is your first time.

How Does It Start?

Here is what's happening: A girl has two ovaries, each of which can house thousands of eggs. An egg is released from one of the ovaries during the menstrual cycle, and it starts its journey down the fallopian tube into the uterus, also known as the womb. One fallopian tube connects each ovary to the uterus.

Hormones encourage the uterus to add more blood and tissue to its inner lining before the egg even leaves the ovary. This is to prepare it for a baby. But don't panic—this doesn't mean you're having a baby.

If the egg is not fertilized by sperm through sexual intercourse, then the egg is mostly just passing through. The uterus no longer requires the additional blood and tissue, thus the blood exits the body through your vagina when the egg is not fertilized. And this is how your period happens.

Typically, a period lasts two to seven days. A new egg is released as the cycle restarts about two weeks after the previous period.

What Is the Best Period Indicator?

When your first menstruation will occur is difficult to predict. However, a white or yellowish vaginal discharge may appear in the few months prior to your period.

The age of the first menstrual cycle is thought to be influenced by a variety of factors, including

- nutrition
- exercise
- genetics
- race
- body mass
- geography (northern climates vs. southern climates)
- family size, composition, and income
- stress and illness

The average age a girl gets her first period is between 12 and 15 years old (Nall, 2019).

You cannot control when your first period will start, so the only thing you can do is wait and try to be informed and prepared. It is extremely difficult to predict when you'll get your first period. Speak to your parents, a counselor, an older sibling, or a doctor if you are anxious about your first period.

What Will It Be Like?

Every girl has a different experience with their period. Periods might differ in length, regularity, and heaviness. While some have very heavy periods, other females have extremely light periods.

Some people experience minor bleeding during their first menstruation. It could start out gradually, with some brown discharge or spots, before turning red.

Others experience a sudden start to their period with bright red blood appearing immediately. Both scenarios are normal. Blood from the period might be brown or deep red in color. Additionally, some people may pass tiny blood clots.

Although some females experience little to no discomfort, having a period might feel comparable to experiencing vaginal discharge. Typical symptoms include

- lower abdominal cramping
- breast sensitivity
- lower back pain
- nausea or diarrhea
- dizziness

Ibuprofen or any other over-the-counter painkillers can be used to treat the majority of these symptoms because they usually pass quickly. Lower back or abdominal pain might be relieved by placing a heating pad or a hot water bottle on these areas.

But we'll talk more about this in Chapters 5 and 6.

How Frequently Do Periods Occur?

Periods may be inconsistent and irregular throughout the first few years following a girl's first period. However, they usually start to happen more regularly over time.

Although the precise length varies from individual to individual and period to period, the average girl gets her period every 28 days. In any given year, the cycle's length can vary by as much as a week.

What Signs Should I Watch For?

Some people experience a sudden start of their periods, but those who are not menstruating may have premenstrual syndrome (PMS) in the days before their menstruation.

PMS symptoms can include

- acne
- stomach bloating
- discomfort in the breasts
- backache

- constipation
- diarrhea
- fatigue (feeling more worn-out than usual)
- feeling especially sensitive or agitated
- cravings for food, especially sweets
- white or clear vaginal discharge

To avoid being totally unprepared when your period starts, you might find it useful to keep a "period kit" in your bag. We'll discuss this later on.

Can I Get Pregnant?

The quick answer? Yes. Any time sperm comes in contact with the vagina, pregnancy is possible.

In general, it is safe to believe that most women who have periods are able to become pregnant.

The beginning of the first menstrual cycle typically indicates ovulation (the process of your egg making its way from the ovary to the uterus through the fallopian tube), and ovulation signifies the possibility for pregnancy. However, during the first couple of years after the first period, both menstruation and ovulation can be irregular, making fertility prediction challenging.

Still, don't take this lightly. It is natural through puberty to start having sexual feelings. But if you do, talk to a trusted adult about it. Your friends, who most likely have zero or unreliable experience with sexual interactions, are not reliable advisors.

Will I Lose Too Much Blood?

First of all, you need to be aware of a fact that was probably never taught to you in school: Only around 50% of menstrual fluid contains blood.

During periods, women typically shed 70–80 ml of fluid and only 35–40 ml of blood per cycle (MM, 2020). This is about equal to the size of a juice box. I know that might seem like a lot, especially when you wake up with a filled pad. But unless you are going through three or four pads per hour, there's no need to worry about your blood loss.

Will I Always Get Periods?

Although it won't last the rest of your life, you'll probably have a period for a while.

Up until menopause, the majority of women will continue to experience menstruation. When the hormones that increase to start your first period begin to decline, menopause sets in. This symbolizes the end of menstruation and the natural reduction in fertility.

Usually, menopause starts between the ages of 45 and 55.

Menopause is thought to have occurred when a complete year has passed without a period. So, since we are years away from this, let's continue to learn how to have healthy and manageable periods.

UNDERSTANDING THE MENSTRUAL CYCLE

Your body uses your menstrual cycle as one of its monthly pregnancy preparation strategies. Since you can use this knowledge to help avoid pregnancy, manage any period symptoms you are currently having, and recognize when there may be a problem, it is crucial to know how the process works.

What Is a Normal Period Cycle?

Normal bleeding can vary; some girls have brief, light periods, while others have longer, heavier periods. Over time, your cycle may also change.

The characteristics of regular menstrual bleeding are as follows:

- Your cycle lasts 3–8 days.
- Every 21–35 days, you get your period again (measured from the first day of one period to the first day of the next month).
- The amount of blood lost overall for the duration of the period is about 2–3 tablespoons

(35–40 ml), although various fluid discharges can make it appear to be more (*Menstrual Cycle Basics*, n.d).

An Outline of the Menstrual Cycle

There are various phases in the menstrual cycle. Every girl's cycle progresses at a slightly different rate which can change over time.

- **Days 1–5**: Day one of the cycle is the first day of menstrual flow. Although the average length is five days, it can extend anywhere between three and eight days. Usually, the first two days are when bleeding is most intense.
- **Days 6–14**: After the bleeding ends, the endometrium, which is another name for the uterine lining, starts to get ready for the chance of becoming pregnant. The blood and nutrients replenish the uterine lining, which thickens.
- **Day 14–25**: Around day 14, an egg leaves one of the ovaries and starts traveling through the fallopian tube to the uterus. This is called ovulation. Fertilization is possible if sperm meets an egg in the fallopian tube or uterus at this time.
- **Days 25–28**: If the egg isn't fertilized or implantation didn't take place, hormonal

adjustments tell the uterus to get ready to release its lining. The egg then fades away and is shed with the lining through your period. On the first day of monthly bleeding, the cycle starts over.

How Can I Track My Cycle? When Do I Ovulate?

You can learn more about your cycle by simply keeping track of it on a calendar along with information about your flow and symptoms. Record the beginning and ending dates of your period, the bleeding, any discomfort or other symptoms (such as bloating, breast pain, etc.), and any changes in your mood or behavior that you encountered. You will be able to recognize trends in your cycle or any abnormalities after a few cycles. Don't worry—you'll get the hang of it. Try keeping a "menstrual diary" or use your own calendar. Numerous apps are also available to assist you in keeping track of your period.

There are a few ways to determine the timing of your own menstrual cycle in addition to simple calendar tracking. Cervical mucus testing and basal body temperature tracking are two techniques you can use to test if you are ovulating, and they can be used individually or in combination.

Cervical Mucus

Your cervical canal's lining cells produce mucus. Over the course of your cycle, this mucus's consistency changes. When you're fertile, the mucus adapts to a structure and thickness that allows the sperm to get to your egg. It will be transparent, abundant, and flexible when you are most fertile. This mucus is commonly referred to as egg white cervical mucus. The mucus is sticky, opaque, and inflexible if you are not fertile.

How Can I Test My Cervical Mucus?

You can better understand your cycle by keeping an eye on the changes in the thickness and volume of your cervical mucus. You can do this by using toilet paper to wipe and inspect your discharge both before and after peeing. Observe and note the color and consistency of your mucus; it may be clear, hazy, white, or yellowish, and it might be sticky or elastic. This means you are in your fertility window and close to your period.

Basal Body Temperature

Your basal body temperature is your body temperature when you are sleeping. Usually, it is tested right after a night of rest. As soon as you start moving about, your temperature gradually rises.

So, how does the basal body temperature ovulation tracking technique work?

It takes a few months of daily tracking with this technique to identify the precise patterns occurring in your body. Ovulation-related hormonal changes cause a modest shift in your body temperature. Your body temperature before ovulation typically ranges between 36.2 °C and 36.5 °C (97.7 °F and 97.16 °F). Your body temperature will rise by at least 0.5 °C (or 0.7 °F) the day after ovulation—36.7 °C to 37.1 °C or 98.06 °F to 98.78 °F, for example—and remain at this level until menstruation (*Menstrual Cycle Basics*, n.d).

Cool, right?

To use this technique, take your body temperature as soon as you are awake and after at least six hours of sleep. This entails taking your temperature before getting out of bed and before consuming any food or drinks. Every day, take your temperature around the same time. You might need to set an alarm if you like to sleep late on the weekends.

You will require a unique "basal body temperature" thermometer, which is sold at pharmacies. You may not have to record the reading right away because some thermometers have a memory function that saves the previous value. On the day following ovulation, you'll notice the temperature rise by half a degree.

MAKING A PERIOD KIT

Believe it or not, this was one of my favorite things to make when packing my bag for high school. Making a period kit can be fun, and most of all, it makes you feel more secure knowing you'll be prepared.

Since our periods can be off by a day or two even when we track it, it's always good to be prepared. So, in this section, we'll learn how to make a period kit for home or school.

How to Make a Period Kit

Making a period kit is quite simple. You can ask your mom or a responsible adult to help you and accompany you to the store or pharmacy to get the essentials for your kit. Here are the steps:

- **Step 1**: First, you'll need a small pouch or sack —something around the same size as your pencil case.
- **Step 2**: Add three to five pads, tampons, or menstrual cups—whatever you're most comfortable using. You'll need to add more than

one since you'll probably need to change at school if your period indeed starts. You should also add pantyliners for spotting or light flow days.

- **Step 3**: Pack an extra pair of underwear just in case your period starts and your underwear gets stained, which leads us to step four.
- **Step 4**: Add a small plastic/zip lock bag for stained underwear.
- **Step 5**: You'll want to add some feminine wipes as well as they will help you to feel clean when you change pads or underwear.
- **Step 6**: You can also add hand sanitizer just in case there's an unfortunate situation with no soap! You can never be too prepared.
- **Step 7**: Though this is optional, it never hurts to add a few painkillers to your kit. Cramps can cause a huge cramp in your day, and maybe a menstrual pill is all you need to save the day. You can also add a small snack or comfort food like a chocolate bar if you want.
- **Step 8**: You're all set! Zip it right up and put it in your backpack.

Here's a helpful tip: Whenever you use something from your kit, be sure to immediately replace it when you go home! This will help you be prepared for the next month just in case you forget to repack your kit before then.

What Do I Do if I Don't Have My Kit?

So what should you do if you don't have your period kit and that pesky little cycle arrives when you least expect it? Don't panic. Here's what you can do instead: You can always ask a very close friend, your teacher, the school nurse, or guidance counselor for an extra pad. It's important that you don't feel embarrassed about such things. Every girl and woman goes through this, and as you grow, you'll learn that nobody is more supportive than a girl helping another girl with a period crisis.

However, if you're in a situation where you can't ask for help, there's an easy fix to that, too. You can use tissue paper or a handkerchief. I know it sounds weird, but it will only be temporary until you can get a sanitary napkin (pad) or a tampon.

Take a handful of tissue paper or a handkerchief, fold it into a thick rectangle, and carefully place it in the crotch of your underwear. This won't last for long, so be sure to get a pad or tampon as soon as possible. But until then, you'll be just fine. Be sure to pull your underwear firmly up if you use either of these methods.

Easy peasy!

Your period years can be frustrating, aggravating, and sometimes embarrassing. But you can be the boss of your own cycle!

PERIOD PENNINGS

Let's reflect!

Getting our period can be a weird time in our lives, and making preparations can be just as crazy. Write about it!

1. How do you feel about starting your period?
2. What's an extra essential that you might put in your period kit?
3. I think my comfort food for my period will be...

Segue: The next chapter talks about taking care of your body when you have your periods.

5

PERIOD CARE

H ave you started your first period and don't know what to do first? Let's help you understand everything about this red-hued world.

WHAT TO USE

You're going to need to use something to absorb the menstrual blood when you start your period. There are various items available. To determine what is ideal for you, some experimenting may be necessary.

Typically, girls will utilize one or more of these items:

- pads (or sanitary napkins)
- tampons

- menstrual cups
- period underwear
- panty liners

These allow you to go on with your normal day when on your period.

Pads

Pads, often known as sanitary pads, are small strips of material that you attach to your underwear. Some have "wings," or flaps, which fold under the sides of your panties to prevent leaks and stains.

There are numerous variations of pads, including

- super
- slender
- overnight
- scented
- maxi
- mini

How to Use Pads

Even if you have a light flow, you should change pads every three to four hours. Changing frequently reduces the growth of bacteria and eliminates odor. Here's how you use it:

- You press the pad into the crotch of your underwear after removing the paper strip covering the stickiness.
- Using the adhesive strip on the back, put the pad inside your underpants.
- If the pad has wings, you should wrap those around the crotch of your underwear.
- Throw away used pads after wrapping them in toilet paper. The toilet can become clogged if you flush used pads or wrappers.

How Do I Choose the Right Pad?

Every girl is different, and this includes the way her body responds to menstruation. This is just one of the reasons behind the wide variety of sanitary napkin options on the market.

Your preference is particular to you because it is influenced by things like your skin type, body type, and flow. Here are some things to think about:

- adequate absorption
- duration and flow
- material of pad (if you have allergies)
- lifestyle

Tampons

The tiny cotton plugs known as tampons are designed to fit inside your vagina and absorb menstrual blood. Some tampons include an applicator to make inserting the tampon easier, and some tampons are applied with your finger. The end of a tampon has a string that makes it simple to draw out.

How to Use Tampons

There are various "sizes" (absorbencies) of tampons, including light, regular, and super. At this stage, it's advisable to use tampons with applicators.

- Ensure your hands are clean and you are in a comfortable position. You can sit on the toilet with your legs apart, squat, or raise one leg.
- Insert the tampon inside your vagina using the applicator.
- You'll feel more at ease inserting a tampon if you're relaxed. The tip of the tampon or applicator can also be coated with a small amount of lubricant. If you're experiencing problems, ask a trusted adult who has used tampons (such as your mother, sister, or another trusted adult) to demonstrate how to insert the tampon.

- Changing your tampon every four to eight hours is recommended. Never wear a tampon for longer than eight hours. Tampons can be worn overnight, but make sure to put them in right before bed and take them out as soon as you wake up.
- A string is attached to tampons on one end. Pulling the string carefully will allow you to remove the tampon.
- Do not flush used tampons; instead, wrap them in toilet paper and dispose of them in the garbage.

Menstrual Cups

Menstrual cups are little bell- or bowl-shaped items made of soft plastic, silicone, or rubber. The cup is inserted into the vagina and is used to collect menstrual blood. The majority of cups are reusable; you simply empty them as needed, wash them, and then use them once again. Other menstruation cups are disposable and can be thrown away after one use or period cycle.

How to Use Menstrual Cups

Despite their size, most individuals cannot feel cups once they are inside the vagina.

- Wash your hands and make yourself comfortable. You can sit on the toilet with your legs apart, squat, or raise one leg.
- Use your fingers to move the cup inside your vagina after narrowing it with a squeeze or fold. To determine how to squeeze and where to position your cup, refer to the instructions that came with it.

If you're relaxed, inserting a cup into your vagina will be more comfortable. If you're having problems, ask someone you can trust to demonstrate how to insert it into your vagina (such as your mother, sister, or another trusted individual).

- Some cups are inserted high in your vagina close to your cervix, and others should be in your vagina's lower region; again, check the instructions on the packaging to be sure where and how to insert yours. Take out your cup and try again if it's uncomfortable or not in the right place.
- A menstrual cup is worn continuously for eight to 12 hours, or until it is full.
- Some menstrual cups feature a tiny stem you can pull to remove it. Others can be taken out

by wrapping a finger around the rim, applying pressure, and tugging it out.

Period Underwear

Similar to regular underwear, period underwear has extra layers of cloth to absorb menstrual blood while you are having your period. For days with light, medium, or heavy menstrual flows, there are various types of period underwear. Period underwear can be worn on its own as well as with a menstrual cup or tampon.

How to Use Period Underwear

Once you're bleeding, wear your period underwear. You may wash your period underwear in the washer the same way you wash the rest of your underwear. The perfect way to wash your period underwear is described in the care instructions that come with them.

You might need to change your period underwear more frequently than once per day if you have a strong flow or are wearing light-flow underwear, or you can use a tampon, pad, or menstrual cup for more protection from leaks and stains.

Panty Liners

Panty liners are essentially tiny variations of pads used to stop stains and maintain clean underwear. Panty liners are designed to absorb regular vaginal discharge, unanticipated light menstrual flow, light spotting, and stains at the start and end of periods. For added security, panty liners can be worn with tampons and menstrual cups.

How to Use Panty Liners

Panty liners aren't usually used for a heavy flow, but here is how they are generally used:

- Panty liners are worn inside underwear similarly to pads, and they have a sticky strip on the underside to hold them in place.
- The crotch of the underwear needs to be covered and fastened with a panty liner inserted vertically.
- If a panty liner gets too wet, it needs to be changed right away.
- At night, avoid using panty liners. To lessen the danger of infection, they should be replaced as frequently as possible.
- Avoid using scented panty liners because they may make you itchy and uncomfortable. Use organic cotton without scents instead.

Which Period Protection Is Right for Me?

The answer to this depends on you! Consider your needs and lifestyle to determine what will work best for you. It also helps to experiment with several products or ask a friend or family member what they like.

During your period, it's normal to utilize different stuff at various times. Tampons might be used in the daytime and pads at night, for instance. While wearing a tampon or cup, you can also use period underwear, a pad, or a panty liner as additional protection in case of leakage.

Some individuals believe that wearing a cup or tampon is more convenient and comfortable because they are hidden and you typically can't feel them.

Others prefer period underwear or pads since they don't want to insert anything into their vagina or even because they find them to be more comfortable than tampons or cups. However, you can't wear these in water, so if you're on your period and plan to go swimming or participate in sports, use a tampon or a cup.

Tampons and pads are examples of items that are popular due to their convenience of use. These are typically simpler to locate in stores as well. Others choose reusable protection, such as cloth pads, menstrual cups, or period underwear, since it's more cost-effective and environmentally friendly.

Use of scented douches, vaginal deodorants, or scented tampons or pads might cause irritation or infection. Some people are concerned about the scent of their period, but it's unlikely that anyone will be able to recognize that you're on your period. Simply remember to change your pads, tampons, period underwear, or cups frequently and you'll be good to go!

WHAT TO WEAR

We might think that when we're on our periods, we should pad up (no pun intended) with layers and layers of clothing to prevent visible staining. But this is not so. In fact, that might put you at more risk of getting infections due to the increased growth of bacteria.

Instead, be comfortable yet safe when dressing.

It's never simple to pick out stylish clothes that are also comfortable, and it's even more difficult when you're on your period. We are very mindful of what we should avoid during that time, but we do give careful consideration to what to wear—something that is both fashionable and comfortable—around that time of the month.

While it's true that comfort is vital during periods, you can't let the excitement of dressing up be taken away by your periods, can you?

We are still functional human beings despite the fact that our female reproductive systems occasionally cause many of us dreadful, intolerable, terrible pain and just make us generally uncomfortable. This implies that wearing actual clothing—as opposed to sweatpants—is necessary to get through the day. The difficulty, however, lies in finding comfortable clothing that can be worn every day.

Here is a list of great comfortable yet stylish clothing options that you can wear when having your period.

Leggings or Jeggings

Yes, jeggings or leggings worn with a cute top can be your look. They are comfortable yet significantly less casual than your sweatpants. They function exactly like jeans or pants, but they're considerably cozier. They are flexible, breathable, and very fashionable. Therefore, if you don't already own a pair of leggings or jeggings, I urge you to get some right away.

Jumpsuits

A single piece of clothing can be heavenly, and jumpsuits are always in style. They are not only comfy and stylish, but they also effectively hide your pad lines from the outside. When worn with the appropriate accessories and footwear, they look quite fashionable and are incredibly simple to wear.

Shirt Dress/T-Shirt Dresses

The shirt dress, which is just like a shirt but long enough to be a dress, can be one of your most comfortable options. They are really comfortable, simple to wear, and informal. Perfect for nights out with your girls and when you want to look stylish but dress casually.

Palazzos

Palazzos are adaptable bottoms with lots of room for your legs to breathe, and they can be worn with practically anything. Isn't that incredible? When you're on your period, your clothing should leave you feeling carefree, and this garment does just that.

Maxi Dress

Maxi dresses are always a good choice. Maxi dresses are highly recommended because they hide any bloating, which keeps you from feeling self-conscious. It is simple to put on and feels comfortable all day!

High-Waisted Clothing

The most common problem seen by women during their periods is bloating. Despite the fact that it is normal, it feels odd, and women feel forced to conceal it. High-waisted jeans are the ideal bottoms in this situation because they will conceal your bloated stomach and prevent you from feeling uncomfortable. To nail the look, pair your high-waisted jeans with crop tops and a cute pair of shoes. Who said you can't look good when you're feeling bad?

Shrugs

Shrugs are a great layering piece when you're on your period because they're not only light and loose, but they also assist in hiding pad lines. Additionally, they essentially save the day if you by chance get your clothes stained. They are simple, cozy, and completely trendy.

Soft Clothing

A soft cashmere sweater that makes you feel like a cloud is engulfing you is without a doubt the way to go when all you want is some warmth and comfort when on your period. Nothing is greater than receiving tenderness and warmth, even from an artificial item like clothing.

Sweatpants

Recall how I said that sweatpants are not the only comfy clothes for periods? They aren't, but nothing is more calming or pleasant than letting your blood flow in a pair of sweatpants. Some people might be self-conscious about leaving home in sweats, but they are a perfect weekend outfit and can still be very chic for school or going out.

SELF-CARE

Self-care is the best care. Until you're old enough to marry a partner who will bring you chocolate and ice cream on your period, it's best if we learn how to take care of ourselves for now.

Always make an effort to take a break to care for your physical and emotional well-being, especially when you're on your period. Because your body is working so hard throughout your period, it's crucial that you pay attention to what it and your emotions are trying to tell you.

However, I understand that it can be challenging to decide what to do when you're experiencing the emotional ups and downs of your period. To help make it simpler for you, I've included some of my all-time favorite self-care techniques so that you may try them out for yourself:

- Shower or take a warm bath.
- Attempt meditation or a form of art.
- Take a walk to get some fresh air.

- With the supervision of an adult, you may need to take pain medication.
- Dress comfortably and wear underwear.
- Eat some menstruation-friendly food (more on this in the next chapter).
- Get lots of rest.
- Use a heating pad or hot water bottle.
- Drink a lot of water.
- Choose period products that are right for you.
- Do something enjoyable for yourself.
- Discuss your feelings with your family and friends.
- Focus on your accomplishments and favorable attributes.
- Play your preferred music.
- Cut back on your screen time.
- Keep a journal.

How Do I Deal With Cramps?

When your body is shedding the uterine lining, you may feel this process through what is referred to as cramps, and they can be painful. You might be able to get relief by

- following the directions on the package when taking over-the-counter medications such as ibuprofen (Advil) or naproxen sodium (Aleve)

- putting a heating pad or wrap on your lower back or stomach and covering it with a cloth
- taking a warm bath

Speak to a responsible adult if your cramps are so bad that you feel sick, can't get out of bed, or are unable to go about your daily activities. The medical name for painful menstruation cycles brought on by uterine contractions is dysmenorrhea. Recurrent pain is referred to as primary dysmenorrhea, whereas reproductive system issues are the cause of secondary dysmenorrhea. Both are treatable. They can give you pain-relieving tabs like Tylenol or Ibuprofen. They may need to take you to the doctor so you can talk about your symptoms. In other instances, excruciating cramping could be a sign of an underlying illness like endometriosis.

PERIOD STAINS ARE OKAY

Yes, they are. They will happen, sometimes at the right time when no one is around, and sometimes someone will have to point it out for you. I can't count the number of times I've had someone tap me on my shoulder and whisper, "Your clothes are stained," in my ear. Sometimes, even men!

The point is, as girls, there might be at least one time in our lives that we get a period stain, and that's okay.

But there are ways we can try to avoid them.

Overnight Pads

Compared to ordinary pads, overnight pads are more absorbent. Therefore, utilizing them could aid in stopping leaks that cause staining. One should be adequate for the whole of the night, but it all depends on your flow. Depending on how you sleep, you can try putting an extra pad in the front or rear of your underwear if you have a very heavy flow. Keep in mind that a longer pad is ideal. Another great trick is wearing these pads during the day if you have a heavy flow.

"But they are overnight pads!"

They are, but who will know? Wearing an overnight pad on your heavy days can help prevent leakage.

Use a Panty Liner With Tampons and Cups

If you are a tampon or menstrual cup person, you can wear a panty liner in your underwear to prevent staining in case of leakage.

Change Your Pad, Tampon, or Cup

Before going to bed, going home from school, or hitting the road, put on a new pad or insert a fresh tampon. Once you've been wearing them for a couple of hours, you should change them for health reasons as well as to avoid leakage.

Period Underwear

Period underwear is the answer if your period is approaching or if you simply want an extra layer of incredibly comfortable protection.

Period underwear is as comfy as your everyday intimates and can be as absorbent as three tampons. If you'd like, you may add a pad or panty liner for extra protection, but be careful to allow your vagina breathing space at all times.

Wear Appropriate Clothing

If you use pads, it would probably be best to wear full undergarments rather than thong-like underwear. This way, your pad won't be able to shift out of place. No matter the type of underwear you wear, ensure your pad is attached correctly in your underwear or that your tampon or cup is inserted properly. Shifting is possible if they are not worn properly, which can lead to stains.

REMOVING PERIOD STAINS

So what happens if you do manage to develop a stain? Do you throw out the clothes and pants? No. Although period stains can be annoying, there is nothing shameful about them because, despite our best attempts, menstrual blood can occasionally leak. The good news is that you can get rid of the stain yourself rather than paying a dry cleaner and hoping your favorite pair of jeans hold up. I've compiled a list of techniques and tricks for getting rid of period stains from your clothes as if they never happened in the first place. Here are six typical items you can probably find in your home that you can use to get period stains out of your clothes.

Ice Water

Never attempt to remove a menstrual stain with hot water. While a warm, soothing bath or steaming shower can help with cramps, it will also make it harder to remove a period stain from your clothes. Ice cold water is your ally when it comes to removing period stains, and it makes a great base before using other remedies.

All-Purpose Stain Remover

There is something for everyone, including products like OxiClean or Clorox as well as natural options. Apply or spray your selected solution, let it sit for 10 minutes to soak, and then rinse with cold water once more. Try hydrogen peroxide if your clothing is lighter in color.

White Vinegar

Although white vinegar can sometimes have a strong odor and taste, many people vouch for its cleaning abilities. It's up to you whether you use vinegar alone or vinegar mixed with a little soap or detergent to treat the stain.

Lemon Juice

The natural acidity of lemon can be used as a secret weapon to remove even the worst period stains. Give the stain five minutes to soak after applying fresh lemon juice. Rub the juice into the stain with a moist towel then rinse with cold water.

Salt

Regular table salt can be a great tool to get stains out of darker clothing. Similar to how salt can magically transform stale movie theater popcorn into a delicious delight, it has the power to get rid of difficult stains and bring your garments and linens back to their former glory.

Baking Soda or Dissolved Aspirin

Assuming that none of the first five approaches were successful in removing these remarkably tough stains, don't lose hope yet! You might be able to remove the stain by using a harsher product, such as crushed aspirin or baking soda. Combine cold water and baking soda to make a paste then apply the mixture to the fabric and gently rub it in.

Also, remember to give each method a good soak, around 30 minutes, before washing it in cold water. Try this and you're all set! You have your lovely dress for another day!

PERIOD PENNINGS

Let's reflect!

Periods can be a menace to girls, but there are always tips and tricks to make them a little more manageable. Let's write about it!

1. The thing I dislike most about my period is…
2. I use/want to use a period self-care method like…
3. I want to be more positive about…because…
4. Are you confident to wear your favorite outfits when you're on your period? If yes, list some ways you feel confident. If no, talk about what kind of outfit you'd like to put together for period days.

_____

Segue: The next chapter talks about what you should eat during your periods.

6

WHAT SHOULD YOU EAT?

Periods can be uncomfortable, and you may experience backaches, stomachaches, or cramps, all of which may accompany the bleeding. If you choose your food wrong, these problems may be aggravated further. Therefore, it is important to practice mindful eating.

In this chapter, I'll show you how to maintain your body and regulate your hormones with food.

Enjoy this meal planning tool to assist you in choosing foods that will support your body's needs throughout each menstrual phase.

WHAT TO EAT BEFORE YOUR PERIOD

Period symptoms can be very unpleasant, and if you've ever questioned why these symptoms appear in a more severe way one month but become much easier to manage the next, keep reading.

Hormonal fluctuations, which are the primary cause of our monthly cycles, are also responsible for well-known (and, yes, bothersome) period symptoms including PMS, mood swings, bloating, and cramps. These symptoms, however, can become severe if your hormones are out of balance. Did you know that what you eat even a day before your period can increase or decrease period cramps? Keep reading to learn more.

Down to the Good Part

Remember when we talked about ovulation which occurs about seven to 14 days before your period? Your progesterone levels increase and your estrogen levels fall during this phase. This means that your mind and body are likely to feel less energetic and be inclined to slow down. You might even experience some sadness or drowsiness.

Strong cravings will cause you to feel hungry more frequently throughout the day. Because of this, it's crucial to have healthy snacks on hand that help your body feel better rather than making cramps, cravings, and bloating worse.

It's actually more necessary to concentrate on foods to avoid than to think about what you should eat during this phase. Reduce the number of processed foods and refined sweets you eat in general. They might not have an impact on your physical health, but they may change your hormone levels and make you more irritable.

Here's what to eat:

- Eat good fats! For hormones to change smoothly, your body requires fats. Olive oil, avocados, and nuts are all excellent choices for healthy fats.
- Your body will produce more progesterone if you add sesame seeds, which are high in zinc, and sunflower seeds, which are high in vitamin E, to smoothies, salads, or breakfast bowls.
- Maintaining a high iron level will help you feel better and have more energy. Include iron-rich foods like almonds, peas, beans, and legumes in your diet to aid with brain fog as well.
- Minimize salt intake as much as you can because salt causes you to retain more water, which increases bloating.

- Your body is naturally attempting to remove excess estrogen during this phase, and whole grains (not refined) like quinoa, buckwheat, or brown rice can help in this process.
- Choose roasted or baked veggies with onion and garlic, such as cauliflower, cabbage, parsnips, radishes, celery, and cucumber, as side dishes for your meals.
- Stay hydrated! Focus on drinking enough water and avoiding sodas and other sugary beverages. Make a nutritious lemonade with fresh mint and ginger and sip chamomile or peppermint tea at night to unwind your body and mind.
- To prevent bloating and bowel irritation, eat fiber-rich fruits and nuts, including almonds, apples, figs, apricots, and pears. These are ideal to keep on hand as nutritious snacks all day. Choose these over a candy bar.

Most, if not all, of the foods listed here are excellent to eat during your period also. But ever heard the saying, "Prevention is better than a cure?" Be mindful of what you eat during ovulation, and you'll have a smoother period.

WHAT TO EAT DURING YOUR PERIOD

Although it's vital to always feed your body for hormonal health, concentrating on particular foods during your menstrual phase can assist to balance your hormones and manage potential discomfort and cramps. It's not all that different from the previous section, but now we'll focus on specific nutrients that you need during your period.

Nutrients Important for Menstruation

During menstruation, estrogen and progesterone are at their lowest levels in order to shed the uterine lining which leads to bleeding. Thus, it's important that you get a lot of iron and vitamin B12.

Iron is a crucial part of hemoglobin, which is a red blood cell protein that transports oxygen throughout the body. Iron is a nutrient that can be found in food organically, in some types of foods with added iron, or in supplement form.

Vitamin B12 is equally important for blood cell formation and energy during this period. In order for red blood cells to operate and nerves to function properly, vitamin B12 is essential.

Foods That Have the Necessary Nutrients

During your menstruation cycle, it's crucial to maintain a balanced diet with enough protein, carbohydrates, and fats to support your hormones as well as concentrate on foods that are high in iron and vitamin B12.

Chicken and fish are excellent sources of iron that helps to replace blood lost during your period. You can also choose non-animal sources of iron, such as peas, beans, and almonds.

To aid in the production of new red blood cells and lessen any tiredness and nausea you may experience during your period, you should also pay attention to meals rich in vitamin B12. Cheese, fish, and eggs are a few foods that are abundant in vitamin B12. Additionally, there are plant-based sources of vitamin B12, such as nutritional yeast and fortified breakfast cereals. You can also grab foods such as

- dark chocolate (which is rich in iron and magnesium)
- lentil and beans (high in iron, protein, and zinc which helps reduce cramps)
- fruits and vegetables
- omega-3–rich foods (flaxseed and flaxseed oil, walnuts, chia seeds, soybean, yogurts, and plant-based milk)

- water (a lot of it)

Food plays a critical role in development, growth, metabolism, reproduction, and mood, all of which depend on appropriate hormonal balance and function.

Cravings

You're not alone if you crave chocolate cake even though your body would much rather have the nutrients from an apple. The additional hunger and desires you may experience before or throughout your period have valid scientific explanations.

During your period, hormones like progesterone and estrogen cause serotonin (the brain hormone that makes you feel good) to decline. We may appear more agitated, frustrated, or annoyed when serotonin levels are low. Cravings for foods high in carbohydrates and sugar before your period are linked to changes in the levels of these hormones.

So, what can you do to best appease these cravings? Planning is essential. In this manner, you are prepared to provide your body with beneficial nutrition from foods like homemade muffins, seasonal fruit, or dark chocolate that is rich in antioxidants. Planning ahead is better than having these cravings suddenly strike while you are unprepared.

WHAT TO AVOID EATING DURING YOUR PERIOD

Similar to how some foods can lessen period symptoms, others can make them worse. These are typically foods that result in bloating or inflammation.

We are lured by unhealthy snacks because many girls are unable to manage their cravings, which can be unpredictable and difficult to overcome. However, if we can find healthy substitutes for unhealthy snacks, you might be able to satisfy your cravings and feast on your favorite foods at the same time! Therefore, you might want to examine your food intake and make some adjustments if you had or are currently experiencing a difficult period.

Spicy Foods

If you enjoy fried foods and ready-made snacks, you might be compelled to eat something spicy. Avoid eating hot and salty food because too much salt will make you retain water, which could make you feel bloated.

Refined Grains

Like other processed foods, refined grains lose some of their nutritional value during processing. They start to interfere with normal appetite management and blood sugar levels as a result, so consider eating whole grains rather than processed pasta or bread.

Coffee

Every morning, you might enjoy a steaming mug of tea or coffee. Maybe in a few years, it'll be impossible for you to wake up without it! However, you should try to avoid this habit during your period. Refrain from drinking that cup of coffee and continue to stay as hydrated as possible.

Fatty Foods

Do you want to go on a binge-eating spree of burgers and fries and down a whole bottle of soda by yourself? Even though it might sound tempting, you should avoid eating meals heavy in fat because they have a negative impact on your hormones. They cause irritation and add to period pain. Therefore, it is advised to stay far from these foods when you are menstruating.

Processed Food

You might enjoy eating a lot of chips and crackers in one sitting, but since they are a main source of salt in your diet, it is important to limit these foods to help reduce your intake of salt.

Alcohol

Although alcohol is not a part of your diet right now, in a few years when you're old enough to drink alcohol, remember this little tip: Alcohol can make you dehydrated which can cause headaches and lead to bloating. Additionally, it may result in digestive problems like diarrhea and nausea.

Red Meat

Prostaglandin—which is "compounds in the body made of fats that have hormone-like effects [that can] include uterine cramping and increased sensitivity to pain"—levels in red meat are high (Nall, 2020). Your body creates prostaglandins during menstruation to aid in uterine contraction and, ultimately, menstrual flow. However, cramps are a result of excessive prostaglandin levels. Because red meat is high in prostaglandins, it is advised to steer clear of it since it'll worsen cramps.

Sugar

While eating sugar in moderation is acceptable, eating too much of it might result in an energy spike followed by a crash. This can make you feel worse. Watching your sugar consumption can help control your mood if you frequently experience moodiness, sadness, or anxiety during your period.

Foods You Have Trouble Tolerating

Even though it might seem obvious, if you have food intolerances, you should always avoid such items, especially when you're on your period.

Despite your lactose intolerance, you might pamper yourself with a milkshake once in a while. However, it's crucial to avoid the items that can cause problems for your health when you're on your period. Eating these meals may result in nausea, diarrhea, or constipation, which will only make your discomfort during a painful period worse.

While some meals can help you feel better during your period, others can make your symptoms worse. Your individual symptoms and food sensitivities will have a big impact on the foods you decide to eat or stay away from.

EXERCISING DURING PERIODS

Do you want to put your running shoes away completely at the idea of exercising while on your period? You're not alone.

Many people neglect their workouts when on their periods for a variety of reasons. However, there's really no justification for skipping a workout because of your period. In fact, exercising while menstruating has its benefits.

Benefits of Exercising on Your Period

Exercise continues to be good for your body and mind even during your period. Actually, maintaining a workout pattern can help relieve some of the usual problems related to menstruation.

You may experience fatigue and a lack of energy during the period phase of your menstrual cycle because, as we know, progesterone and estrogen levels are at their lowest.

Therefore, skipping exercise won't help you feel better or conserve energy. Use the week of your period as a chance to attempt some new workouts rather than stopping all activities. In truth, exercise can boost your mood by boosting endorphin synthesis (also known as "feel-good hormones") and lowering stress, sadness, and pain. But getting even mild activity during your period can help with symptoms like

- pain
- cramps
- bloating
- depression
- mood swings

- irritability
- fatigue/nausea

Here are five other detailed benefits of exercising during your period.

Reduce the Symptoms of PMS

Regular aerobic workouts may help reduce your feelings of weariness and mood swings if you experience them during your cycle and in the days preceding your period.

Engage Your Endorphins

Endorphins are brain-produced hormones that have soothing and pain-killing effects on the body. Exercise can improve your mood and make you happier since it causes a natural endorphin rush. The endorphin production and exercise "rush" are two of the key advantages of exercising when on your period. Endorphins are a type of natural painkiller, so when they are released during exercise, you might experience a reduction in discomfort.

Gain Greater Strength and Power

Due to low levels of female hormones, the first two weeks (ovulation to the first day of period) of the menstruation cycle may allow you to enjoy greater improvements in strength and power.

Improve Your Mood

Your mood and circulation will both improve if you exercise. Exercise can also help with period-related headaches, backaches, and cramps.

Combat Painful Periods

If you have dysmenorrhea—or painful periods—you are all too familiar with how difficult menstruation can be. The great news is that you might be able to lessen these symptoms with exercises like brisk walking.

Best Exercises to Do on Your Period

If you happen to bleed a lot throughout this time, the initial days of menstruation may be the most painful. This is why you should prioritize doing mild exercises and motions.

Find the one that you like the most and whichever one works most effectively. Here are some suggestions for exercising while on your period.

Walking or Other Light Cardio

Reduce the intensity of your aerobic or cardiovascular exercise or cut back on how much you undertake. Think about doing some gentle aerobics, walking, or short bursts of exercise. Consider saving more intense types of exercise for later in your cycle since your lungs perform better then.

Low-Volume Strength Training and Power-Based Exercises

These exercises should be included because there may be a strength improvement during this phase. In fact, this is a fantastic time to perform longer flow workouts that combine aerobics with stretching exercises.

Yoga

Yoga might help you calm your body and possibly lessen symptoms like cramps, breast soreness, and muscular exhaustion and pain in the two to three days prior to your period.

Stretching

Tossing and turning in your bed is not as effective as doing simple home stretches. If performing other workouts causes you greater pain, consider stretching and taking deep breaths to relax your body's muscles.

Feel free to keep up with your typical exercise schedule if your period is not causing you any pain. Just be aware of the changes your body goes through at this time. Give yourself a pause or reduce the intensity if you notice that your body isn't functioning as it typically does.

Exercises to Avoid

There are some workouts that might be better avoided while you're on your period. In general, you should lower your exercise intensity and stress levels during your period. This merely means to scale back a bit on your workout rather than stopping altogether.

When you are menstruating, your body may not respond well to intense or extended activity. You don't have to stop your regular exercising as a result, but proceed cautiously. So, you might want to avoid lifting heavy weights or running for extended periods of time.

Lastly, stop what you're doing and take a break if you experience unexpected exhaustion, nausea, or an increase in pain or discomfort. If these signs appear, stop immediately. Be mindful of your body.

Last Thing

Your body and mind will benefit from regular exercise. There is no scientific justification for skipping your workouts while you are on your period. In fact, there is proof that exercising during your period can be beneficial (Lindberg, 2018).

The conclusion is as follows: Maintain your exercise routine but reduce the intensity, especially if you are feeling exhausted. Change up your routines, give yourself more time to recover, and respect your limits.

PERIOD PENNINGS

Let's reflect!

We might have already known that nutrition and health are important, but on your period? Isn't your period supposed to be the time of the month when you are allowed to treat yourself or break the rules a little?

Well, maybe, but the consequences can be hard. So, let's write about it.

1. What do you usually eat while on your period?
2. Fun task: Create a period menu for your next cycle (you may include a guilty pleasure snack).
3. Do you normally exercise? If yes, how will you incorporate your routine to help during your period? If not, how can you start a routine for your period?

Segue: The next chapter talks about changing feelings, something that you hide from everyone but weighs heavy on your heart.

7

TALKING ABOUT YOUR FEELINGS

A lot goes on inside the head and heart of a teenager. It's almost like their entire brain chemistry gets rewritten. You must have felt this happen to you, too. New friendships, weird crushes... You have a different world that you have built up inside your head, don't you? In times like this, you really need someone dependable to talk to. Who might that someone be?

PMS

A lot of people don't realize this, but "PMSing" is an actual thing. It's actually an acronym for premenstrual syndrome, and as the 'pre' suggests, it happens before your menstrual cycle. In other words, it's all the symptoms (except the actual bleeding) that we get during our period, only before the actual period.

However, in theoretical terms, premenstrual syndrome, or PMS, describes changes to behavior, physical health, and mood that

- develop between the time of ovulation and the beginning of your period (about two weeks before your period)
- last up to a few days after the start of your period
- continuously appear each month
- have an effect on routine tasks and daily life in some way

PMS is a highly common issue. About 20% of women of reproductive age have PMS, and for about 48% of them, the symptoms are severe enough to cause problems with daily activities (Raypole & Higeura, 2022).

Regardless of what some individuals may believe, PMS is a serious condition that can significantly interrupt everyday life and bring both physical and mental discomfort. But not to worry, the rest of this section will give descriptions of PMS symptoms along with advice on how to cope with them and get help.

Symptoms of PMS

While PMS frequently has mild to moderate symptoms that have little to no influence on day-to-day activities, symptoms can also be serious enough to have a detrimental effect on your everyday routines and general well-being.

You will regularly experience PMS symptoms before each menstrual period if you have it. Even though you might just experience a few of the symptoms listed here, most women's PMS frequently has at least a few symptoms.

Emotional Symptoms

Mood, emotional, and behavioral changes brought on by PMS may include:

- anxiety, agitation, or feeling tense
- unusual irritation and anger
- change in appetite, including increased appetite and food cravings, particularly for sweets
- changes to sleep habits, including exhaustion and difficulty falling asleep
- a depressed or melancholy attitude that may be accompanied by tearfulness or abrupt, uncontrollable crying
- quick mood swings and emotional outbursts

- having trouble focusing or remembering things

Physical Symptoms

You may also experience certain physical signs of PMS, such as:

- stomach pain and bloating
- aching and enlarged breasts
- acne
- constipation
- diarrhea
- headaches
- muscle pain and backaches
- unusually high sensitivity to sound or light
- a peculiar clumsiness

Although PMS cannot be cured, there are things you may take to lessen your symptoms.

Treatments

Try the following tactics to see if they can help you with your mild to moderate PMS symptoms:

- To reduce belly bloating, drink plenty of fluids. This includes tea that may relieve cramping, such as chamomile and red raspberry leaf.

- Consume a diet that is well-balanced and rich in fruits, veggies, and whole grains.
- If your body is particularly susceptible to the effects of alcohol, coffee, sugar, and salt, you might want to reduce your intake of these substances.
- To aid with cramping and mood problems, consult a healthcare provider about trying supplements like folic acid, vitamin B6, calcium, and magnesium.
- Consider consuming more vitamin D-rich foods or supplements or spending more time in natural light.
- Get seven to nine hours of sleep every night to help with fatigue relief and enhance general well-being.
- If you can, try to engage in at least 30 minutes of physical activity each day.
- Exercise can help relieve symptoms of anxiety and depression in addition to bloating and cramping.

Take a moment each day for self-care, which can include things like exercise, rest, alone time for hobbies, or socializing.

Additionally, over-the-counter drugs and therapies can lessen the physical manifestations of PMS. Options include:

- aspirin, ibuprofen, or acetaminophen for headaches and muscle pain or ibuprofen for stomach cramps
- heating pads or wraps that are applied to your abdomen to ease cramping
- cognitive behavioral therapy (CBT) or other therapy modalities can help you learn new strategies to reframe and cope with painful thoughts and feelings if you experience severe mood symptoms that interfere with your everyday life
- ask your parents and/or a doctor to assist you with any form of treatment

CHANGING FRIENDSHIPS

We might admit that as teenagers, we tend to prioritize socializing with our peers over spending time with our families. We might feel like our friends make us feel more welcomed and understood.

Teens from the same social class, ethnic origin, and with similar hobbies frequently become close friends. Teen friendships broaden to include similarities in attitudes, beliefs, and shared activities, whereas childhood friendships typically focus on shared activities. The common theme in teen friendships is a shared interest in learning. Close, personal, and self-disclosing interactions with friends, particularly for girls, help in the exploration of identities and the definition of one's sense of self-worth.

Why Do Friendships Change in Teenage Years?

Some of us might stay close with our childhood friends all the way through your teenage years and even into adulthood—that's the whole point of "best friends forever," after all. However, there is a possibility of growing apart, and here are a few reasons why.

You Have More Control

The children of your parents' friends made obvious candidates for playmates when you were young. You'll start looking for connections that are wholly your own as you get older.

New Classmates and Schools

You will undoubtedly make new friendships as you leave the safety of elementary school and move into middle school and high school.

Pursuing Mutual Goals

Friendships are frequently built around shared interests in the preteen and adolescent years. It's common for your friendship groups to change as you grow as a person and uncover your passions.

Although each of the above reasons is an absolutely reasonable (and healthy) explanation for switching up one's social circle or for gradually drifting away from long-standing friendships, this doesn't mean you have to let go of your old friends completely.

The factors influencing friendships will never go away, but your love and devotion to a friend might never change. If it is changing, however, don't panic or be afraid to let go. You'll both need space to grow as individuals and figure yourselves out along the way.

Just let it flow!

Unhealthy Friendships

Friendships can become unhealthy at times. Unhealthy friendships can have an adverse effect on mental health, including low self-esteem, stress, anxiety, and a sense of being emotionally or physically exhausted.

Because it can be challenging to let go of a cherished connection, you may maintain unhealthy friendships for longer than you ought to. However, if warning signs are ignored, significant harm and pain may have already been done by the time the friendship reaches its breaking point. It's critical to recognize the indicators that it's time to say goodbye when friendships that initially appeared to be strong and long-lasting need to end for a variety of reasons. Some of these signs are

- drama—a lot of drama
- control (dictating friendship)
- continual fighting
- peer pressure (pressuring you into something you're uncomfortable with)
- they treat you badly
- they treat other people poorly

So, down to the hard part: How do you end a friendship?

Well, the key is to be honest. Tell them that you are uncomfortable and you need some space. Growing up, you'll notice that you will need to do this... a lot. It's good for not just your mental health, but your life, too. So, start practicing now.

ROMANTIC FEELINGS

Teenagers can learn a lot from romantic relationships about communication, feelings, compassion, identity, and even sex in some cases. These lessons are crucial for stimulating growth, resiliency, and happiness in adolescents, as well as serving as a basis for lasting relationships in adulthood.

Having a romantic partner during adolescence can increase your confidence. Young people are more content with themselves when relationships are defined by intimacy and excellent communication. Young people appreciate the comfort, intimacy, and support they get from romantic relationships. Despite the notion that conflict within intimate relationships gets worse with age, young people have more disagreements with their parents and classmates than they do with their love partners (Act for Youth, n.d). For young couples, spending time doing things that both partners enjoy is important. Relationships frequently end when this aspect of connection is absent.

Relationships and Romance in Preteens and Teenagers

A significant developmental milestone is having romantic relationships.

These interactions arise along with all the other physical, social, and emotional changes that occur during adolescence. They are associated with how preteens and teenagers discover their identities, privacy, independence, and body image. These relationships may also allow some young individuals to explore their sexual orientation.

You, and occasionally your entire family, may experience numerous emotional ups and downs as a result of romantic relationships. However, these emotions are developing your capacity to care, share, and form close bonds at a deeper level.

When Preteen and Teenage Love and Romance Begin

There is no set age at which you should begin romantic relationships, but around the following ages, changes frequently occur:

- You may begin to exhibit greater independence from your family and an increased interest in friends between the ages of nine and 11.

- By the ages of 10 to 14, you may begin to experience feelings of attraction toward some peers.
- From the ages of 15 to 19, romantic relationships can take on a significant role in your social life.

Children usually don't show any interest in romantic relationships until they are in their teens. Some young people decide to prioritize their studies, sports, or other pursuits, which is usually advised.

First Crushes

You may harbor one or more crushes before you start dating.

The first sign of romantic emotions is a crush. It has to do with viewing someone else as beautiful or ideal. This might reveal a lot about the traits in others that appeal to you. This is completely natural and a part of growing up.

Even if you try to resist them, you may not be able to make your feelings go away. In times when this happens, be careful and smart with your actions and feelings. Talk to a trusted adult, an older sister, or a family member you can trust.

DEALING WITH HARASSMENT

Bullying and harassment are abusive ways to treat others.

Bullies and harassers make hurtful remarks, gestures, threats, or physical acts. They attempt to injure, exclude, offend, or humiliate others.

Bullies and harassers occasionally engage in sexually explicit language or behavior; this is called sexual bullying or sexual harassment.

Examples of sexual harassment and bullying include:

- making sexually explicit jokes, remarks, or actions to the victim
- spreading sexism-related rumors about the victim (in person, by text, or on social media)
- uploading sexually explicit messages, images, or videos of the victim
- capturing and sharing explicit photos and videos of the victim
- asking someone to take their own naked photos ("nudes")
- offering to have sex or soliciting sex
- a sexually suggestive touch or grab

Online and offline sexual harassment and bullying are both possible. However, sexual bullying and harassment are not acceptable in any setting, and the victim of bullying or harassment is never to blame.

Inform a responsible adult if you or somebody you know is suffering through this. If the first adult you tell doesn't put a stop to it, continue notifying other adults until the harassment and bullying end.

Here are some suggestions that may work in the majority of cases:

- **Realize the truth.** Remind yourself that you are not to blame. No matter what the harasser may claim, a victim "asking for it" is not a thing. You deserve to feel secure.
- **Demand that they stop.** Inform them that you don't approve of their behavior when it occurs the first time. Be brief, relaxed, and clear. Then make your exit. That will suffice in some circumstances, but not always. They might continue. They may even ignore your request, make fun of you, or bother you again.
- **Tell a grown-up.** You shouldn't attempt to tackle this on your own. Speak to a parent, coach, teacher, counselor, parent of a friend, a relative, or a doctor. At first, mentioning it

could feel awkward, but don't let it deter you. Find another adult to speak with if the one you're talking to won't listen or provide assistance.

- **Report it.** Inform a responsible adult if this occurs at home or school. To protect you, the majority of educational institutions have a sexual harassment or bullying policy. They must be aware of the situation in order to assist you and prevent it from happening again.
- **Get assistance.** Consult a therapist or counselor if you're experiencing stress, depression, anxiety, or insomnia as a result of this. They can assist you in coping with the stress and recovering from it.

Bullying

When someone is victimized by a person or group, it is called bullying. Bullies may make fun of individuals they view as different or believe don't belong.

Bullies may make fun of people for a variety of reasons, such as:

- appearance
- behavior (how someone acts)
- religion or race
- public standing (whether someone is popular)
- sexual orientation (such as being gay, lesbian, or transgender)

How Can I Help?

If you are being bullied or know a person who is, there are several things you can do to stop it:

- **Again, tell a responsible adult**. Bullying is frequently dealt with by adults in positions of authority, such as parents, teachers, or coaches, without the bully ever knowing how they learned about it.
- **Turn your back on the bully and leave**. Bullies enjoy provoking their victims. You're sending them the message that you don't care by ignoring them or leaving.
- **Avoid physical contact**. If you try to fight a bully, you run the risk of getting hurt and into trouble. Work through your rage in another way, like through exercise, talking, or writing.
- **Develop your confidence**. Practice how to react to the bully both verbally and nonverbally. Make an effort to feel good about yourself.

- **Discover your (real) friends**. Inform your friends if you have been the target of rumors or gossip bullying so they can make you feel protected and secure. Avoid being alone, particularly if bullying is often near you.
- **When you notice friends or others being bullied, speak up for them**. Your acts make the victim feel reassured and could possibly put an end to the bullying.
- **Participate in the anti-bullying or anti-violence programs at your school**. Another way you might be able to resolve your conflict with a bully is through peer mediation.

And if you're not a victim but you know someone who is being bullied or harassed, do these things just the same. Speak up for them, don't be silent, be confident and helpful, and be a real and true friend.

Be awesome and loving, girls!

TALKING TO YOUR PARENTS

You may speak more often with your friends than with your parents. Regardless of if you and your parents get along well, this is normal.

Even so, it's beneficial to have a parent's assistance, counsel, and support.

Opening up could initially seem uncomfortable, especially when discussing certain topics. If you haven't had a heart-to-heart in a while, it could feel harder to start the conversation. Being honest with your parents is a wonderful idea. In actuality, it is very helpful.

Here are some suggestions for topics to discuss:

- **Talk about ordinary issues**. Make it a practice to discuss routine issues from your day with your parents. Share your successes, a pleasant memory from your day, a grade you're proud of, or a humorous joke a friend cracked. Talking with each other promotes intimacy and increases enjoyment. In this manner, it is easier to talk about a big issue you are having when you need to.
- **Discuss a challenge you are facing**. Some children may believe that by talking about an issue, they will worry or upset their parents. But whether it's a big or small concern, parents can handle being informed. If they appear concerned, it just signifies that they are sympathetic and care about you.

- **Discuss your feelings**. You can learn more about yourself by talking about your feelings. It supports effective emotional management. A parent may be the ideal person to confide in. After all, they are rather familiar with you. With them, you may be really honest.
- **Take part in activities that both of you enjoy**. When you make time to spend with your parents, talking to them is simple. Invite your parents to join you for a walk, game, sport, cooking activity, or watching TV shows you both enjoy. Spending time together enables you two to unwind, have fun, and feel close. That makes it simple to open up and communicate with them—about anything or about nothing at all.
- **Discuss an issue that worries you**. Tell your parents what's on your mind if you have any concerns. Even talking about a concern might decrease its impact. Parents can also give you advice on how to deal with your worries, and you'll feel more equipped as a result.

Tips on How to Get the Conversation Rolling

Even though at times it might seem really difficult—especially when you know you are the one who has messed up or done something you shouldn't have—it's best to know how to talk to your parents. These are the times when you must learn to talk to your parents without tantrums and tears. You just need to bite the bullet and talk. So, here are a few tips to get the conversation rolling:

- Try to write down what you're going to say in advance.
- There might never be a "right time" to start a discussion, so try to do so when you're at your calmest.
- To feel more prepared, practice the talk with a friend or a counselor.
- Select a quiet area where you won't be disturbed and feel comfortable speaking.
- You don't need to know every solution. It's okay to say, "I don't know," and let your parents help you work it out.
- If things become too stressful, take a break. The discussion may need to span several days or weeks.
- If you're feeling particularly anxious, have a friend or sibling at your side for support.
- Find a time that works for everyone to talk.
- It will be easier to keep the conversation on topic if you stick to one or two primary points.

Perhaps you need to inform your parents that you failed an exam. Perhaps you're anxious or scared about something. Or maybe you want to share a personal story about a close friend or family member. However, you can't be sure of their response or how telling them will feel until you just do it.

But we should always remember that our parents have seen it all, or if not *all*, at least a version of it. And most importantly, they love us. So, yes, going to a friend might seem easier, but especially now, make it a habit to build a trustworthy relationship with your parents.

It will make your teenage years much easier.

PERIOD PENNINGS

Let's reflect!

Wooh. That was a ride. Growing up can be hard, weird, and funny. But what do you think about the entire process? Write it down!

1. I want to talk to my parents about…
2. I love my friends and I wish to maintain our friendship. So, I will…
3. If you notice a friend is being bullied or harassed, what will you do?

4. Overall, what is your honest opinion about the entire process of growing up? Write a journal entry about it, then try to make journaling a habit.

_____

Segue: This is not the end of your journey to discover adolescence. Pick up our next book, _Ladyish_, for learning more about your body, your life as a teenager, and the best way to reach adulthood gracefully.

CONCLUSION

Girls, this is a time of growth.

It can be scary, but it can also be an exciting experience once we have the correct knowledge, support, network, and relationships. Though we might start to see changes in the way we express our feelings, this is completely normal, and we shouldn't feel compelled to "feel" emotional just because we are females. However, when you do, let it all out, and find the best way for you to cope with it. Always remember that this is all due to puberty and hormones. In this stage, hormones will be crazy, driving our emotions, minds, and bodies all over the world and back. But remember you are the master of your own body and heart, so let them flow naturally but don't lose yourself in the process.

While this stage of life only lasts a few years, we all know that our periods stay with us for a bit longer, so we ought to know how to care for ourselves during this period and find the best way to deal with symptoms and cramps. Periods can be a menace, but they are something we have to live with, so let's not allow our periods to beat us, but let's beat our periods instead!

And lastly, in this stage of growing up, you will find new friends, lose old friends, and crushes will come and go. But remember that your family is constant, so try to strengthen your relationship with your parents now. If you already have a strong relationship with your mom and dad, aunt or uncle—whomever it may be, make talking with them about every topic a habit. Your future self will thank you for it.

So, as we go, let's love ourselves and others and grow into the wonderful, beautiful, magnificent young women we are destined to be. I cherish each and every one of you (even if I don't know you personally), and I feel that I have formed a bond with each of you!

If you have enjoyed reading this book as much as I enjoyed writing it, please leave a review and share it with your friends!

So, until next time—stay sweet, my girls!

REFERENCES

Acne. (2020, January 9). Cleveland Clinic. https://my. clevelandclinic.org/health/diseases/12233-acne

Anzilotti, A. (2019, October). *Tampons, pads and other period supplies*. TeensHealth. https://kidshealth.org/en/ teens/supplies.html

Barendse, M., Cheng, T. & Pfeifer, J. (2020 April 30). *Your brain on puberty*. Frontiers. https://kids.frontiersin. org/articles/10.3389/frym.2020.00053

Barnes, M. (2021, October). *Talking to your parents or other adults*. TeensHealth. https://kidshealth.org/en/ teens/talk-to-parents.html

Barrell, A. (2022, April 28). *At what age do girls stop growing?* Medical News Today. https://www.medicalnewsto day.com/articles/320668#takeaway

BBC. (2014, September 17). *Private parts*. https://www. bbc.co.uk/science/humanbody/body/articles/lifecycle/ teenagers/sexual_changes.shtml

Bravier, Y. (2020, October 25). *What to know about Puberty.* Medical News Today. https://www.medical newstoday.com/articles/156451

Chaplin, T. & Aldao, A. (2012, December 12). *Gender differences in emotion expression in children.* National Library of Medicine. https://www.ncbi.nlm.nih.gov/ pmc/articles/PMC3597769/

Coyle Institute. (n.d). *Teenage hormone imbalance: When to talk to a doctor.* Coyle Institute. https://coyleinstitute. com/understanding-teenage-hormone-imbalance/

Dovi, A. (2021, June). *Sexual harassment and sexual bullying.* TeensHealth. https://kidshealth.org/en/teens/ harassment.html

Dowshen, S. (2015, October). *All about puberty.* Kids-Health. https://kidshealth.org/en/kids/puberty.html

Duchesne, K. (2020, January 13). *Real talk: How to get period stains out of underwear and clothing.* Byrdie. https://www.byrdie.com/how-to-remove-period-stains-4774965

Emotional changes that occur during puberty. (n.d). Menstrupedia. https://www.menstrupedia.com/arti cles/girls/emotional-changes

EUSci. (2020, April 9). *Why do humans—and so few other animals—have periods?* https://eusci.org.uk/2020/04/

09/why-do-humans-and-so-few-other-animals-have-periods/

Ferguson, S. (2019, July 16). *16 foods to eat (and some to avoid) during your period.* Healthline. https://www.health line.com/health/womens-health/what-to-eat-during-period#takeaway

Friendship changes in the teenage years. (2021, September 16). Life Insight. https://life-insight.com/friendship-changes-in-the-teenage-years/

Gavin, M. (2018, July). *Cellulite.* TeensHealth. https://kidshealth.org/en/teens/cellulite.html

Gavin, M. (2019, June). *Dealing with bullying.* Teens-Health. https://kidshealth.org/en/teens/bullies.html

Gavin, M. (2021, January). *Should I gain weight?* Teens-Health. https://kidshealth.org/en/teens/gain-weight.html

Hirsch, L. (2021, November). *Acne.* TeensHealth. https://kidshealth.org/en/teens/acne.html

How do I use tampons, pads, period underwear, and menstrual cups? (n.d). Planned Parenthood. https://www.plannedparenthood.org/

Hyde, P. (2016, August). *Hair removal.* TeensHealth. https://kidshealth.org/en/teens/hair-removal.html

Jaspan, R. (2022 January 31). *What to eat during your period to help you feel your best.* Very Well Fit. https://www.verywellfit.com/food-for-your-period-5216405

Kabotyanski, K. & Somerville, L. (2021, February 2). *Puberty: your brain on hormones.* Frontiers. https://kids.frontiersin.org/articles/10.3389/frym.2020.554380

Khona, M. (2022, January 17). *16 effective skin care tips for teenagers.* SkinRaft. https://skinkraft.com/blogs/articles/skin-care-tips-for-teenagers

Kinonen, S. (2020, December 23). *The science of beauty: The complete guide to body hair.* Allure. https://www.allure.com/story/body-hair-guide

Lindberg, S. (2018, September 17). *Can you exercise on your period?* Healthline. https://www.healthline.com/health/exercise-during-period#exercises-to-avoid

Lyness, D. (2021, September). *Talking to your parents.* TeensHealth. https://kidshealth.org/en/kids/talk-parents.html

Marcin, A. (2019, March 13). *Height in girls: When do they stop growing, what's the median height, and more.* Healthline. https://www.healthline.com/health/when-do-girls-stop-growing#growth-and-puberty

Marcin, A. (2022, March 22). *Navigating puberty: the Tanner stages.* Healthline. https://www.healthline.com/health/parenting/stages-of-puberty#takeaway

Marhol, A. (2018 December 7). *Exercising during your period: Benefits and things to avoid.* Flo. https://flo.health/menstrual-cycle/lifestyle/fitness-and-exercise/exercising-during-period

Mayo Clinic Staff. (n.d). *Cellulite.* Mayo Clinic. https://www.mayoclinic.org/

Menstrual cycle basics. (n.d). SOGC. https://www.yourperiod.ca/normal-periods/menstrual-cycle-basics/

M.M. (2020, February 24). *Menstrual blood loss. What's normal?* Menstrual Matters. https://www.menstrual-matters.com/bloodloss/

Moods: helping pre-teens and teens manage emotional ups and downs. (2021, May 13). Raising Children Network. https://raisingchildren.net.au/pre-teens/

Nall, R. (2020, January 20). *Everything you want to know about prostaglandins.* Healthline. https://www.healthline.com/health/prostaglandins

Nall, R. (2019, April 15). *What to expect from your first period.* Healthline. https://www.healthline.com/health/first-period#pregnancy

Osborn, C. (2019, October 10). *How to hit puberty faster.* Healthline. https://www.healthline.com/health/how-to-hit-puberty-faster#in-girls

Pattnaik, C. (2021, May 6). *These 7 period hacks will ensure you never stain your clothes ever again.* Health Shots. https://www.healthshots.com/intimate-health/menstruation/these-7-period-hacks-will-ensure-you-never-stain-your-clothes-ever-again/

Pickhardt, C. (2010, July 19). *Why there is more emotional intensity to manage during adolescence.* Psychology Today. https://www.psychologytoday.com/us/blog/surviving-your-childs-adolescence/201007/adolescence-and-emotion

Pitone, M. (2020, November). *Stretch marks.* Teens-Health. https://kidshealth.org/

Pratt-Bercaw, J. & Dietrich, J. (n.d). *Breast development.* Texas Children Hospital. https://www.texaschildrens.org/health/breast-development

Pruess, A. (2018, January 25). *What your daughter needs to know about her emotions.* Parents With Confidence. https://parentswithconfidence.com/what-your-daughter-needs-you-to-know-about-emotions/

Puberty: adolescent male. (n.d). Johns Hopkins Medicine. https://www.hopkinsmedicine.org/health/wellness-and-prevention/puberty-adolescent-male

Puberty (female). (2008, July 25). Health Engine. https://healthinfo.healthengine.com.au/puberty-female

Puberty pimples: a guide for teens. (2021, June 1). WMFC Health. https://wfmchealth.org/pediatric-health-care/puberty-pimples-a-guide-for-teens/

Raypole, C. & Higuera., V. (2022, January 28). *PMS: Premenstrual syndrome symptoms, treatments, and more.* Healthline. https://www.healthline.com/health/premenstrual-syndrome#treatment

Relationships and romance: pre-teens and teenagers. (2021, September 14). Raising Children Network. https://raisingchildren.net.au/pre-teens/communicating-relationships/romantic-relationships/teen-relationships

Romantic relationships in adolescence. (n.d). Act for Youth. https://actforyouth.net/sexual_health/romantic.cfm

Roy, T. (2020, October 21). *7 foods to avoid during menstruation.* Zoom. https://www.zoomtventertinment.com/lifestyle/health-fitness/article/7-foods-to-avoid-during-menstruation/670467

Sawyers, T. (2019, January 22). Do stretch marks go away? *Healthline.* https://www.healthline.com/health/stretch-marks#getting-rid-of-them

Sinha, R. (2022, July 27). *Stretch marks in teenagers: How to deal with them.* StyleCraze. https://www.stylecraze.com/articles/stretch-marks-in-teenagers/

Sherrell, Z. (2021, November 25). *What to eat on your period to relieve symptoms.* Medical News Today. https://www.medicalnewstoday.com/articles/what-to-eat-on-your-period

Shkodzik, K. (2018, December 8). *What are panty liners for? Are they good for you?* Flo. https://flo.health/menstrual-cycle/

Smith, J. (n.d.). *What to eat before, during and after your period: A guide.* Ruby Cup. https://rubycup.com/blogs/news/a-helpful-guide-on-what-to-eat-before-during-and-after-your-periods

Summer clothing: Comfort clothes you should wear during your periods. (2019, April 5). Sofy. https://www.sofy.in/blog/tips-tricks/generic-concerns/summer-clothing-comfort-clothes-you-should-wear-during-your-periods/

Villines, Z. (2021, January 26). *First period: Early signs and what to expect.* Medical News Today. https://www.

medicalnewstoday.com/articles/317595#Spotting-vs-period-Whats-the-difference

Young, K. (2015 August). *19 Practical, powerful ways to build social-emotional intelligence in kids & teens.* Hey Sigmund. https://www.heysigmund.com/social-emotional-intelligence/

Your first period. (n.d). SOGC. https://www.yourperiod.ca/normal-periods/your-first-period/